LIST OF CONTRIBUTORS

Dr RJ Atkinson MRCP(UK)
Consultant Physician and Gastroenterologist
Calderdale and Huddersfield NHS Foundation Trust
Huddersfield

Dr GM Hirschfield MA MB BChir PhD MRCP(UK)
Clinical Lecturer in Hepatology
Addenbrooke's Hospital
Cambridge

Dr SC Keshav MBBCh DPhil FRCP
Consultant Physician and Gastroenterologist
Department of Gastroenterology
John Radcliffe Hospital
Oxford

Dr JS Leeds MBChB MRCP(UK)
Honorary Clinical Lecturer in Gastroenterology
Gastroenterology and Liver Unit
Royal Hallamshire Hospital
Sheffield

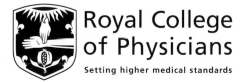
Royal College
of Physicians
Setting higher medical standards

© 2008 Royal College of Physicians of London

Published by:
Royal College of Physicians of London
11 St. Andrews Place
Regent's Park
London NW1 4LE
United Kingdom

Set and printed by Graphicraft Limited, Hong Kong

First edition published 2001
Reprinted 2004
Second edition published 2008

ISBN: 978-1-86016-271-8 (this book)
ISBN: 978-1-86016-260-2 (set)

Distribution Information:
Jerwood Medical Education Resource Centre
Royal College of Physicians of London
11 St. Andrews Place
Regent's Park
London NW1 4LE
United Kingdom
Tel: +44 (0)207 935 1174 ext 422/490
Fax: +44 (0)207 486 6653
Email: merc@rcplondon.ac.uk
Web: http://www.rcplondon.ac.uk/

MEDICAL MASTERCLASS

EDITOR-IN-CHIEF

JOHN D FIRTH DM FRCP
Consultant Physician and
Addenbrooke's Hospital
Cambridge

GASTRO
HEPATOL

EDITOR

SATISH C KESHA
Consultant Physician and
John Radcliffe Hospital
Oxford

Second Edit

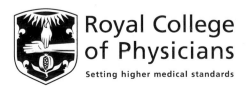

Royal College
of Physicians
Setting higher medical standards

Disclaimer

Although every effort has been made to ensure that drug doses
and other information are presented accurately in this publication, the
ultimate responsibility rests with the prescribing physician. Neither the
publishers nor the authors can be held responsible for any consequences
arising from the use of information contained herein. Any product
mentioned in this publication should be used in accordance with the
prescribing information prepared by the manufacturers.

The information presented in this publication reflects the opinions of its
contributors and should not be taken to represent the policy and views of the
Royal College of Physicians of London, unless this is specifically stated.

Every effort has been made by the contributors to contact holders of
copyright to obtain permission to reproduce copyrighted material. However,
if any have been inadvertently overlooked, the publisher will be pleased to
make the necessary arrangements at the first opportunity.

CONTENTS

CONTENTS

FOREWORD

Since its initial publication in 2001, *Medical Masterclass* has been regarded as a key learning and teaching resource for physicians around the world. The resource was produced in part to meet the vision of the Royal College of Physicians: *'Doctors of the highest quality, serving patients well'*. This vision continues and, along with advances in clinical practice and changes in the format of the MRCP(UK) exam, has justified the publication of this second edition.

The MRCP(UK) is an international examination that seeks to advance the learning of and enhance the training process for physicians worldwide. On passing the exam physicians are recognised as having attained the required knowledge, skills and manner appropriate for training at a specialist level. However, passing the exam is a challenge. The pass rate at each sitting of the written papers is about 40%. Even the most prominent consultants have had to sit each part of the exam more than once in order to pass. With this challenge in mind, the College has produced *Medical Masterclass*, a comprehensive learning resource to help candidates with the preparation that is key to making the grade.

Medical Masterclass has been produced by the Education Department of the College. A work of this size represents a formidable amount of effort by the Editor-in-Chief – Dr John Firth – and his team of editors and authors. I would like to thank our colleagues for this wonderful educational product and wholeheartedly recommend it as an invaluable learning resource for all physicians preparing for their MRCP(UK) examination.

Professor Ian Gilmore MD PRCP
President of the Royal College of Physicians

PREFACE

The second edition of *Medical Masterclass* is produced and published by the Education Department of the Royal College of Physicians of London. It comprises 12 textbooks, a companion interactive website and two CD-ROMs. Its aim is to help doctors in their first few years of training to improve their medical knowledge and skills; and in particular to (a) learn how to deal with patients who are acutely ill, and (b) pass postgraduate examinations, such as the MRCP(UK) or European Diploma in Internal Medicine.

The 12 textbooks are divided as follows: two cover the scientific background to medicine, one is devoted to general clinical skills [including specific guidance on exam technique for PACES, the practical assessment of clinical examination skills that is the final part of the MRCP(UK) exam], one deals with acute medicine and the other eight cover the range of medical specialties.

The core material of each of the medical specialties is dealt with in seven sections:

- Case histories – you are presented with letters of referral commonly received in each specialty and led through the ways in which the patients' histories should be explored, and what should then follow in the way of investigation and/or treatment.

- Physical examination scenarios – these emphasise the logical analysis of physical signs and sensible clinical reasoning: 'having found this, what would you do?'

- Communication and ethical scenarios – what are the difficult issues that commonly arise in each specialty? What do you actually say to the 'frequently asked (but still very difficult) questions?'

- Acute presentations – what are the priorities if you are the doctor seeing the patient in the Emergency Department or the Medical Admissions Unit?

- Diseases and treatments – structured concise notes.

- Investigations and practical procedures – more short and to-the-point notes.

- Self assessment questions – in the form used in the MRCP(UK) Part 1 and Part 2 exams.

The companion website – which is continually updated – enables you to take mock MRCP(UK) Part 1 or Part 2 exams, or to be selective in the questions you tackle (if you want to do ten questions on cardiology, or any other specialty, you can do). For every question you complete you can see how your score compares with that of others who have logged onto the site and attempted it. The two CD-ROMs each contain 30 interactive cases requiring diagnosis and treatment.

I hope that you enjoy using *Medical Masterclass* to learn more about medicine, which – whatever is happening politically to primary care, hospitals and medical career structures – remains a wonderful occupation. It is sometimes intellectually and/or emotionally very challenging, and also sometimes extremely rewarding, particularly when reduced to the essential of a doctor trying to provide best care for a patient.

John Firth DM FRCP
Editor-in-Chief

ACKNOWLEDGEMENTS

Medical Masterclass has been produced by a team. The names of those who have written or edited material are clearly indicated elsewhere, but without the support of many other people it would not exist. Naming names is risky, but those worthy of particular note include: Sir Richard Thompson (College Treasurer) and Mrs Winnie Wade (Director of Education), who steered the project through committees that are traditionally described as labyrinthine, and which certainly seem so to me; and also Arthur Wadsworth (Project Co-ordinator) and Don Liu in the College Education Department office. Don is a veteran of the first edition of *Medical Masterclass*, and it would be fair to say that without his great efforts a second edition might not have seen the light of day.

John Firth DM FRCP
Editor-in-Chief

KEY FEATURES

We have created a range of icon boxes that sit among the text of the various *Medical Masterclass* modules. They are there to help you identify key information and to make learning easier and more enjoyable. Here is a brief explanation:

> Iron-deficiency anaemia with a change in bowel habit in a middle-aged or older patient means colonic malignancy until proved otherwise.

This icon is used to highlight points of particular importance.

> Dietary deficiency is very rarely, if ever, the sole cause of iron-deficiency anaemia.

This icon is used to indicate common or important drug interactions, pitfalls of practical procedures, or when to take symptoms or signs particularly seriously.

GASTROENTEROLOGY AND HEPATOLOGY

Authors:

RJ Atkinson, GM Hirschfield, SC Keshav and JS Leeds

Editor:

SC Keshav

Editor-in-Chief:

JD Firth

1.1 History-taking

1.1.1 Heartburn and dyspepsia

Letter of referral to general medical outpatient clinic

Dear Doctor,

Re: Mr Ben Harrison, aged 68 years

This man has had retrosternal burning pain for many years, usually helped by over-the-counter antacids. However, in the last 6 months his pain has been more troublesome and sometimes unresponsive to the antacids, and he has also developed upper abdominal discomfort. Has he developed a peptic ulcer, or is something else responsible for his dyspepsia?

Yours sincerely,

Introduction

Dyspepsia is an unpleasant sensation in the upper abdomen. If new, it is an 'alarm' symptom in patients over the age of 45 years and requires rapid investigation because of the obvious concern that it is due to a carcinoma of the stomach. The most common cause is inflammation or ulceration of the upper gastrointestinal tract; other causes are listed in Table 1.

It is important to remember that pain or discomfort in the upper abdomen can come from many sources (eg gallbladder and pancreas) and therefore a careful history is essential. Upper abdominal symptoms may also be referred from above the diaphragm, although this is unusual. Young patients (<45 years) are unlikely to have malignant disease and can therefore be investigated non-invasively.

History of the presenting problem

Pain

Dyspepsia pain is most frequently felt in the epigastric region. Ask about the following.

- Duration: dyspepsia lasting for longer than 6 months is likely to be of benign origin.

- Radiation: pain going through to the back is suggestive of a duodenal ulcer or a pancreatic cause; pain radiating to the right upper quadrant or shoulder tip may indicate a biliary cause.

- Relieving or precipitating factors: gastric ulcer pain is typically worst on eating whereas duodenal ulceration is worst between meals and relieved by food; biliary pain may be stimulated by fatty foods; ischaemic intestinal pain usually occurs as food passes down the small bowel and arises some time after a meal. Does the pain come on during activity? It seems unlikely in this case, but angina can sometimes present as upper abdominal pain.

- Nocturnal pain: functional disorders very rarely cause disruption of sleep.

Other symptoms

Key issues to ask about include the following.

- Vomiting: may indicate obstruction. The nature of the vomitus is important: gastric outlet obstruction leads to regurgitation of undigested food, sometimes many hours after it was ingested; haematemesis clearly suggests peptic ulceration.

- Reflux of an acid taste into the mouth: suggests hiatus hernia. Smoking and alcohol history along with caffeine intake are important in those with reflux symptoms as they represent

TABLE 1 **DIFFERENTIAL DIAGNOSIS OF DYSPEPSIA**		
Common	**Less common**	**Rare**
Gastric ulceration/gastritis[1]	Cholecystitis/gallstones	Atypical cardiac pain
Duodenal ulceration/duodenitis[1]	Chronic pancreatitis	Intestinal ischaemia
Gastric carcinoma	Pancreatic carcinoma	
Functional dyspepsia		

1. Testing for and treating *Helicobacter pylori* is of value in these groups.

potentially beneficial lifestyle modifications.

- Early satiety: a significant symptom associated with gastric cancer and therefore needs investigation, but can occur in benign as well as malignant disease. Some patients with peptic ulceration get pain or discomfort on eating, which leads them to stop, and early satiety can also be a feature of functional dyspepsia.

- Abdominal distension or bloating: may suggest a functional cause.

- Change in bowel habit: melaena would indicate the possibility of peptic ulceration, but also neoplasia. Diarrhoea may suggest malabsorption such as found in chronic pancreatitis, which commonly causes pale stools that float (difficult to flush away) or are fatty/oily (steatorrhoea) in addition to epigastric pain.

- Weight loss: how much and over how long? Significant loss of weight increases the likelihood of significant pathology but can also occur with benign disease, in particular if eating causes pain and induces the patient to reduce intake.

> 🔑 Dyspepsia with weight loss necessitates urgent investigation to rule out gastric cancer.

- Episodes of jaundice, dark urine and pale stools: consider biliary disease.

Other relevant history

Medications and alcohol
What remedies have been tried already and how effective were they? The lack of symptom relief with antacids in this case may indicate that acid is not the cause. NSAIDs and steroids can cause peptic ulcer disease. Warfarin and drugs that inhibit platelet function clearly increase the risk of haemorrhage.

A high alcohol intake predisposes to gastritis as it is directly irritant to the stomach. Alcohol excess is also the leading cause of chronic pancreatitis in the UK and a risk factor for cancers of the stomach and pancreas, hence a detailed alcohol history is required in this patient.

Past medical and surgical history
Is there a history of peptic ulcer disease or of gastric surgery? In the past, partial gastrectomy with or without gastroenterostomy used to be performed for bleeding gastric or duodenal ulcers, and there is an increased incidence of stomal ulceration and carcinoma of the stoma following partial gastrectomy.

Does the patient have a history of cardiovascular, cerebrovascular or peripheral vascular disease? Arteriopaths may have ischaemic intestinal pain.

Are there any other serious medical comorbidities? Any major comorbidities may limit the choice of investigation for a patient, eg endoscopy is more risky in the presence of significant cardiorespiratory disease.

Plan for investigation and management
After explaining to the patient that under normal clinical circumstances you would examine him you would plan as follows.

> 🔑 **Key investigations for dyspepsia**
> - Ascertain *H. pylori* status by serology unless previously treated.
> - Endoscopy: allows biopsy and testing for *H. pylori* if indicated.
> - Abdominal ultrasound scan.

Routine blood tests

- Check FBC for evidence of iron-deficiency anaemia.

- Liver function tests: to aid detection of biliary disease.

- *H. pylori* serology, as long as the patient has not had previous eradication therapy.

- Consider measuring serum amylase for pancreatitis if the patient has suffered recent pain.

Endoscopy
Any structural abnormalities can be visualised and biopsied; biopsy of the stomach near the antrum can also be used to help detect the presence of *H. pylori* by commercially available urease tests.

> ⚠️ No matter how likely the diagnosis of a benign cause, a patient over the age of 45 years with new-onset dyspepsia requires investigation with endoscopy to rule out malignancy.

Imaging
Upper abdominal ultrasound scanning allows imaging of the liver, pancreas and biliary tree and is the radiological investigation of choice. It is best used for imaging solid organs (Fig. 1) and gives little information on the stomach and small intestine unless there is marked pathology, eg gastric cancer causing thickening of the stomach wall. Remember that it is not infallible and can miss distal common bile duct stones and minimal changes in the pancreas.

Other tests
If a biliary or pancreatic cause is likely, then CT or MRI scanning may be appropriate. If endoscopy is contraindicated, then a barium meal

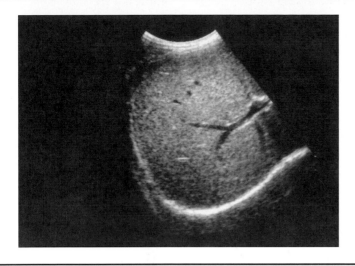

▲**Fig. 1** Normal ultrasound appearance of the liver and bile ducts.

may be performed, but this can miss small lesions and does not allow tissue sampling.

Management

Specific management will depend on the cause. For patients with functional dyspepsia aim for symptom control, which often requires a combination of acid suppression and antispasmodics. Therapies that have been tried include proton pump inhibitors, antispasmodics (such as mebeverine) and antidepressants (particularly low-dose amitriptyline).

1.1.2 Dysphagia and feeding difficulties

Letter of referral to gastroenterology outpatient clinic

Dear Doctor,

Re: Mrs Deborah Finch, aged 67 years

I would be grateful for your assessment of this woman who has noticed increasing difficulty in swallowing over the last 6 weeks. She has a long history of reflux symptoms and uses ranitidine for this. She has also had a stroke in the past. She does not think she has lost any weight but is unsure about this. I am concerned about her symptoms and would value your opinion as to whether they are related to dysmotility or some other problem.

Yours sincerely,

Introduction

Dysphagia means difficulty swallowing and is an 'alarm' symptom that should be investigated rapidly. It may be due to dysfunction in the mouth, pharynx or oesophagus, with the history usually identifying oral problems. Causes are listed in Table 2, but the obvious concern is that it might be due to a carcinoma of the oesophagus or gastric cardia, which should be the working diagnosis until proven otherwise.

Pain on swallowing is known as odynophagia, but although patients may describe this together with dysphagia, it is the latter that is the most concerning.

⚠ Although the patient will often indicate the apparent level of obstruction on the sternum, this correlates poorly with the actual site of blockage.

History of the presenting problem

Related to difficulty in swallowing

- Speed of onset: rapidly progressive dysphagia is suggestive of a malignant stricture, whereas gradual onset of symptoms stretching back over 6 months or more is typical of a benign stricture.

- Problems with solids and/or fluids? Strictures (benign or malignant) usually cause dysphagia first for food (particularly bread and meat) and later for liquids. Dysphagia for liquids (more so than solids)

TABLE 2 DIFFERENTIAL DIAGNOSIS OF DYSPHAGIA		
Common	**Less common**	**Rare**
Benign oesophageal stricture	Pharyngeal pouch	Scleroderma
Oesophageal carcinoma	Achalasia	Motor neuron disease
Oesophageal dysmotility	External compression from	Myasthenia gravis
Stroke	lung lesion	Parkinson's disease
		Multiple sclerosis

often indicates a pharyngeal problem, eg stroke, motor neuron disease. Dysphagia for solids and liquids from the outset is typical of achalasia.

- Is there regurgitation? This may suggest hold up of food in the oesophagus. Nasal regurgitation is associated with neurological causes of dysphagia.

- Pain on swallowing: this occurs in reflux oesophagitis, achalasia, oesophageal candidiasis and herpetic oesophagitis, and also with benign and malignant strictures.

Other symptoms
Any mechanical blockage to the passage of food into the stomach will restrict calorie intake and result in weight loss. Severe and rapid weight loss tends to point to a malignant process.

Is there a history of reflux acidity with an acid taste coming up into the mouth? Chronic acid reflux can lead to oesophagitis with subsequent stricture formation, and patients with gastro-oesophageal reflux disease (GORD) can also develop dysmotility due to chronic acid damage. Epigastric pain may suggest peptic ulcer disease and reflux.

Patients with some neurological diseases can develop dysphagia due to involvement of the upper third of the oesophagus (striated muscle). Stroke with pseudobulbar palsy is the most common, but dysphagia can also be seen in motor neuron disease, multiple sclerosis, Parkinson's disease and myasthenia gravis.

Other relevant history

Drugs
NSAIDs, potassium salts, bisphosphonates and tetracyclines

have all been implicated as causes of oesophagitis and oesophageal stricture formation. Immunosuppressive medications, diabetes mellitus, chemotherapy or HIV infection predispose to oesophageal candidiasis, which may be asymptomatic or cause symptoms of heartburn and dysphagia.

Past medical history
Radiation-induced oesophagitis may occur weeks or months after irradiation treatment for malignancies (eg bronchial carcinoma). Are there any other serious medical comorbidities? These may limit the choice of investigation for a patient, eg endoscopy is more risky in the presence of significant cardiorespiratory disease.

Social history
Alcohol excess and smoking are both risk factors for the development of oesophageal cancer as well as being aspects of lifestyle that could be usefully modified in patients with GORD.

Plan for investigation and management
After explaining to the patient that under normal clinical circumstances you would examine her you would plan as follows.

Routine blood and radiological tests

- Check FBC for evidence of iron-deficiency or other anaemia.

- Electrolytes.

- Renal function (may be impaired due to dehydration).

- Liver and bone function tests (albumin a marker of nutrition).

- Inflammatory markers.

- Haematinics.

- Plain CXR (may show hiatus hernia or carcinoma of the lung leading to dysphagia by external compression).

Investigation of the oesophagus

> **Investigation of dysphagia**
> - Barium swallow (urgent).
> - Endoscopy: biopsy and brushings to exclude malignancy if any stricture is identified.
> - Manometry: consider if endoscopy or barium study negative to exclude achalasia.

> ⚠ No matter how likely the diagnosis of a benign stricture, a patient with dysphagia requires investigation with a barium swallow and endoscopy to rule out malignancy.

Barium swallow This is the most appropriate initial investigation when a patient describes high dysphagia. It allows the site of pathology to be identified and forewarns of pitfalls such as a pharyngeal pouch (Fig. 2), which if unidentified increases the risk of perforation at endoscopy if vision becomes obscured as the endoscope passes through the cricopharyngeus muscle.

If dysphagia is not severe or if a stricture has been previously diagnosed and located (Fig. 3), then endoscopy may be the initial investigation.

Endoscopy Endoscopy allows characterisation of the type and length of a stricture. Any stricture must be brushed and biopsied to exclude malignancy. Dilatation and/or stenting may be performed if a stricture is impassable and dysphagia severe.

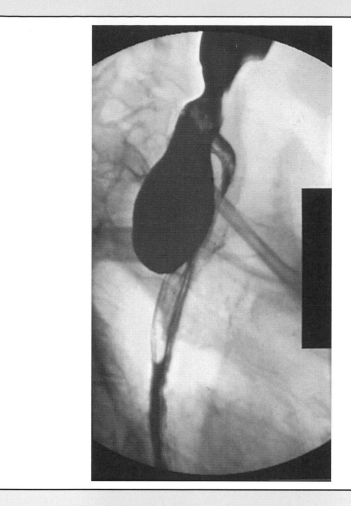

▲ **Fig. 2** Barium swallow demonstrating a large pharyngeal pouch.

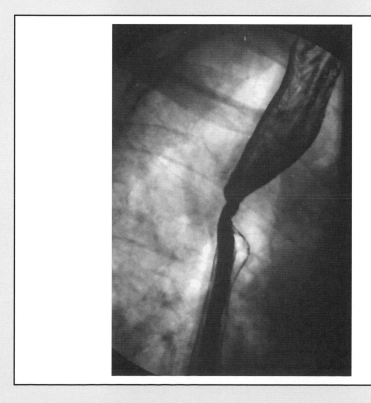

Manometry and pH studies

Oesophageal manometry may be useful in diagnosing a motility disorder (eg oesophageal spasm) if barium swallow and/or endoscopy are normal. It may also provide additional confirmatory evidence of achalasia (hypertensive lower oesophageal sphincter that fails to relax on swallowing) following a suggestive barium study. pH studies can direct therapy in patients with reflux symptoms and can also identify patients with 'silent' reflux.

> Dysphagia without oesophageal narrowing should lead to consideration of dysmotility, which can be identified and classified by manometry.

Other tests

Other investigations may be required in some cases, eg serological tests in suspected scleroderma, electromyography (EMG) in suspected motor neuron disease.

Management

Specific management will depend on the cause identified (Table 2). Patients with neurological causes may require artificial feeding, particularly if the condition is non-reversible and likely to deteriorate over time. Nasogastric tube feeding may be necessary in the short term, but for extended feeding programmes the best option is percutaneous endoscopic gastrostomy.

◄**Fig. 3** Barium swallow showing a benign mid-oesophageal stricture.

1.1.3 Chronic diarrhoea

Letter of referral to gastroenterology clinic

Dear Doctor,

Re: Mr Darren Weaver, aged 24 years

Thank you for seeing this married man with no significant past medical history who complains of a 6-month history of diarrhoea with blood mixed in with the stool. Problems started after he ate a 'dodgy' meal and he assumed that they were infective, but matters have not improved. He has lost some weight and also complains of arthralgia. What do you think is responsible for these problems?

Yours sincerely,

Introduction

This man is most likely to have idiopathic inflammatory bowel disease (IBD), but it is important to exclude chronic infection and to consider other causes of chronic diarrhoea (Table 3). In older patients intestinal neoplasia and paradoxical 'overflow' diarrhoea caused by chronic constipation must not be forgotten, and always check that the patient does actually have diarrhoea, ie increased daily stool volume.

Coeliac disease is common and may present subtly with chronic diarrhoea and vague malaise.

History of the presenting problem

Patients assign their own meaning to technical terms, so always check what they mean by diarrhoea, constipation, 'runs', 'accident', etc.

Relating to the diarrhoea

- Stool frequency and volume: how often, how much and for how long? Be precise: 'How many times have you opened your bowels since you woke up this morning? How many times did you get up last night? Is it a little or a lot on each occasion?' Other markers of severity would be if the patient feels faint or unwell when passing stool, or if there is undigested food in the stool.

- Associated symptoms: ask about urgency, pain on defecation, tenesmus, passage of mucus or pus, bleeding.

- If there is rectal bleeding, is the blood passed freely, sometimes without any stool? Is it mixed

TABLE 3 DIFFERENTIAL DIAGNOSIS OF CHRONIC DIARRHOEA

Type of condition	Diseases/comments
Intestinal inflammation	Idiopathic IBD: ulcerative colitis, Crohn's disease[1] Microscopic/lymphocytic/collagenous colitis NSAID enteropathy Intestinal tuberculosis, which may be clinically indistinguishable from Crohn's disease Radiation enteritis, colitis and proctitis
Chronic infectious diarrhoea	In HIV infection and other immunocompromised individuals: organisms frequently encountered are microsporidia and *Cryptosporidium*; cytomegalovirus and atypical mycobacterial infections may occur. It is debatable whether a specific HIV enteropathy exists as a separate entity Some enteric infections such as giardiasis and amoebiasis may produce prolonged symptoms even in immunocompetent individuals[1] Tropical sprue Whipple's disease *Clostridium difficile*-related diarrhoea is usually acute, but may be chronic and relapsing[1]
Intestinal neoplasia	Intestinal lymphoma may complicate coeliac disease and chronic immunosuppressive therapy Adenomas, particularly secretory villous adenomas of the colon, can produce a secretory diarrhoea Obstructing neoplastic lesions may produce chronic constipation and paradoxical 'overflow' diarrhoea[1]
Malabsorption	Pancreatic insufficiency, eg chronic pancreatitis Coeliac disease[1] Bacterial overgrowth[1] Bile salt diarrhoea due to ileal disease and reduced absorption of bile salts
Systemic disorders and drug-related diarrhoea	Thyrotoxicosis Secretory neuroendocrine tumours, such as carcinoid, phaeochromocytoma, VIPoma Diarrhoea is a frequent side effect of some drugs, such as olsalazine, mycophenolate mofetil, misoprostol, colchicine and antibiotics[1] Factitious/fictitious Laxative abuse

1. Relatively common conditions.
IBD, inflammatory bowel disease; VIPoma, vasoactive intestinal peptide-secreting tumour.

with the stool? Is it only present on the toilet paper when the anus is wiped (suggesting piles)?

- Exclude steatorrhoea: ask if the stool is bulky and light-coloured, floats on the water in the toilet, and/or has an offensive odour.

Other symptoms

- Systemic: in any patient presenting with chronic diarrhoea ask specific questions to determine if there has been weight loss or a systemic response revealed by fevers and sweats. Non-specific malaise, with or without weight loss, is frequently present in uncomplicated ulcerative colitis and coeliac disease. Weight loss, fever, night sweats and malaise are usually prominent in patients with Crohn's disease and intestinal tuberculosis.

- Pain: cramping abdominal pain often accompanies diarrhoea of any cause. Deep-seated abdominal pain should alert to the possibility of Crohn's disease, intestinal tuberculosis and neoplasia. Pain suggesting pancreatitis or cholelithiasis may provide a clue to the cause of steatorrhoea.

Other relevant history

Age is important in that neoplasia is very unlikely in a young patient such as this man. IBD and coeliac disease, on the other hand, can present at any age. Tuberculosis is particularly common in Asia and Africa. The rare condition of Whipple's disease occurs almost exclusively in older men, and microscopic colitis occurs typically in older women.

Apart from a positive family history, there are no known risk factors for IBD, although in some patients it appears to be triggered by an

episode of infectious colitis. The main risks for chronic pancreatitis are excess alcohol use and cholelithiasis, although patients heterozygous for the cystic fibrosis mutation may be at increased risk of idiopathic chronic pancreatitis.

Direct questions are usually needed to address possible endocrine disorders, carcinoid syndrome, HIV disease, travel ('When did you last go abroad? How long were you there? What were you doing? And the time before that?'), diet, and laxative and other drug use. Arthralgia, arthritis, skin rashes and visual symptoms can be associated with IBD.

Plan for investigation and management

Examination of the stool

All patients should have stool examined for bacterial pathogens and for the ova, cysts and adult forms of various parasites. Amoebae may be difficult to detect if a fresh ('hot') stool sample is not examined. If the test is available, estimation of faecal leucocytes is invaluable in distinguishing inflammatory disease from other causes of diarrhoea. In some cases it is necessary to measure the stool volume over a 24-hour period or to estimate faecal fat excretion over a 72-hour period.

> **🔑** Infective causes must be excluded in all cases of chronic diarrhoea.

Endoscopy and imaging

- Rigid sigmoidoscopy: rectal involvement is almost universal in ulcerative colitis, while the rectum may be spared completely in Crohn's disease. Bleeding,

ulceration and a mucopurulent exudate may be seen, although in less severe inflammation there may simply be loss of vascular patterns and a granular friable mucosa. Biopsies should be taken for histological examination.

- Colonoscopy: allows direct visualisation of the entire colonic mucosa and in many cases allows examination and biopsy of the terminal ileum. It should be performed in all patients with suspected colitis or Crohn's disease and may be the most direct way of establishing a diagnosis in other patients (Fig. 4).

- Plain abdominal radiograph: visible dilatation of the large intestine may presage perforation and is an emergency, although this is most unlikely to be seen in an outpatient setting (see Section 1.4.2); pancreatic calcification may help establish a diagnosis of chronic pancreatitis.

Blood tests

Routine blood tests include FBC (anaemia, leucocytosis), electrolytes (hypokalaemia), renal/liver (hypoalbuminaemia)/ bone profile, inflammatory markers, iron/ferritin/folic acid/vitamin B_{12}; clotting screen; anti-tissue transglutaminase antibodies (virtually diagnostic of coeliac disease, although the test may be falsely negative in patients with IgA deficiency).

> **🔑** Raised systemic inflammatory markers are unusual in ulcerative colitis unless the disease is severe, but Crohn's disease can produce a marked systemic response with few clinical signs.

Station 2: History Taking **9**

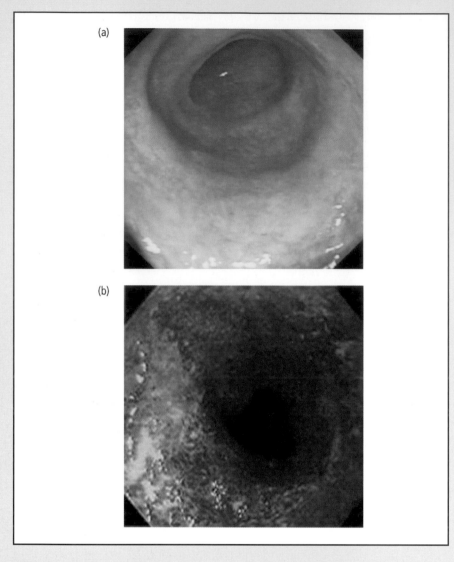

▲ Fig. 4 Ulcerative colitis: **(a)** normal colonic mucosa; **(b)** inflamed colonic mucosa at endoscopy.

⚠ Intercurrent infectious diarrhoea should always be considered, even in patients with known IBD, particularly before starting immunosuppression.

🔑 The management of patients with IBD requires a long-term multidisciplinary approach, including dietitians, specialist nurses, physicians and surgeons.

1.1.4 Rectal bleeding

Letter of referral to gastroenterology outpatient clinic

Dear Doctor,

Re: Mr Richard Venner, aged 56 years

Thank you for seeing this man who has noticed blood in his stools. Over the last 8 weeks he has also developed lower abdominal discomfort and feels that he has lost weight. On examination I thought there might be a mass in the right iliac fossa. He is understandably worried as his mother died of bowel cancer aged 70 years. I would be grateful for your assessment as to the cause of his bleeding and for further evaluation of his abdominal findings.

Yours sincerely,

Assessment and management of nutrition is a key feature of looking after patients with chronic diarrhoea, particularly those with IBD with small intestinal involvement. Iron, folate and B_{12} are absorbed preferentially in different parts of the small intestine and abnormalities may provide clues to localisation of disease processes. In malabsorption due to pancreatic and biliary disease, fat and fat-soluble vitamin absorption are most affected: serum calcium, vitamin D and prothrombin time, which is prolonged by vitamin K deficiency, are informative in these cases.

In rare cases it may be necessary to proceed to test fasting gut hormone profiles to look for abnormal concentrations of gastrin, glucagon and vasoactive intestinal peptide (VIP). The carcinoid syndrome may be diagnosed by increased urinary excretion of 5-hydroxyindoleacetic acid.

Management

Specific management will depend on precise diagnosis. Attention to nutrition is required in all cases of chronic diarrhoeal illness.

Introduction

Rectal bleeding is a common problem and has a wide differential: the most common causes are

---

TABLE 4 DIFFERENTIAL DIAGNOSIS OF RECTAL BLEEDING

Common	Less common	Rare
Haemorrhoids	Colitis (ulcerative colitis or Crohn's disease)	Mesenteric ischaemia
Diverticular disease		Intussusception
Colorectal carcinoma	Colitis (infective)	Volvulus
Anal fissure	Angiodysplasia	Radiation colitis/proctitis
	Arteriovenous malformations	Trauma
		Bleeding disorder
		Portal hypertension with rectal varices

TABLE 5 DIFFERENTIAL DIAGNOSIS OF A RIGHT ILIAC FOSSA MASS

Common	Uncommon	Rare
Ileal Crohn's disease: younger patients with clinical features of inflammatory disease	Appendix mass: abscess, mucocele	Tuberculosis (TB): although TB may cause an ileitis and regional lymphadenopathy, it rarely causes a palpable mass
Caecal carcinoma: older patients with anaemia and subacute bowel obstruction	Ovarian carcinoma[1]	Lymphoma

1. Not in this patient!

Blood seen on wiping only is typical of a perianal cause, whereas blood mixed in with the stool suggests colonic disease.

> ⚠ **Although haemorrhoids may occasionally bleed briskly, such symptoms should not be attributed to haemorrhoids without investigation.**

- How much? Small amounts of bleeding may be caused by anal fissures; large volumes of blood loss require investigation, but even benign causes may lead to substantial haemorrhage.

> 🔑 **Patients often overestimate blood loss because small amounts can discolour the water in the toilet giving the false impression of a large haemorrhage.**

haemorrhoids, colorectal cancer and diverticular disease; other causes are shown in Table 4. The patient's age is an important factor: younger patients are more likely to have an inflammatory diagnosis, whereas those over 55 years have an increased risk of colorectal cancer.

The suggestion of a right iliac fossa mass raises other diagnostic possibilities (Table 5).

> 🔑 **The two main questions to ask about an abdominal mass are as follows.**
> - Is it related to the gut (including liver and pancreas) or another intra-abdominal organ (eg ovary, kidney)?
> - Is it part of a more generalised disease process?

History of the presenting problem

Regarding the rectal bleeding

- Duration: a long history (>6 months) means that the diagnosis is unlikely to be carcinoma.

- When does it occur? Bleeding from haemorrhoids usually coincides with bowel opening, whereas bleeding from other causes may lead to passage of blood at other times.

- What is it like? Bright red blood is commonly seen in distal lesions, whereas dark-red blood may be transported from the proximal colon. Is it malaena, which indicates an upper gastrointestinal tract source or occasionally a caecal lesion?

- Is it seen in the pan, mixed in with the stools or on wiping?

Other symptoms

- Perianal: discomfort or itch may indicate haemorrhoids. Anal fissures may be exquisitely painful: haemorrhoids are not usually painful unless they have thrombosed.

- Abdominal pain: that caused by diverticular disease is typically felt in the left iliac fossa. Cramping pain may occur in colitis. Pain is generally a late sign in neoplasia. Severe pain accompanying bleeding in an ill patient is highly suggestive of mesenteric ischaemia.

- Alteration in bowel habit: any change, particularly to diarrhoea/looseness, is highly significant, especially in the presence of rectal bleeding. This would probably indicate colorectal cancer but is also seen in inflammatory conditions (eg Crohns' disease). A history of chronic constipation is commonly obtained in patients with diverticular disease or anal fissures.

- Nausea or vomiting: these may indicate partial intestinal obstruction, particularly if associated with colicky abdominal pain.

- Anorexia and (particularly) weight loss: these are worrying symptoms, again possibly indicating a neoplasm but also seen in inflammatory bowel disease and intestinal TB, and can considerably pre-date bleeding and the development of an abdominal mass.

- Systemic symptoms: fever may be vague and at best non-specific, but reports of mouth ulcers, arthralgia and gritty eyes are common in patients with Crohn's disease.

- Symptoms of pelvic disease: ask explicitly about urethral discharge and pneumaturia (which means that there must be a fistula between bladder and bowel), and in women also enquire about vaginal symptoms such as discharge.

Other relevant history

Past medical and surgical history
Enquire about the previous diagnosis or possibility of chronic liver disease with portal hypertension, which might result in rectal varices, and also about bleeding diathesis or radiotherapy to the abdomen or pelvis, either of which could lead to rectal bleeding.

Take note of previous cardiovascular, cerebrovascular or peripheral vascular disease, diabetes, hypertension or

hypercholesterolaemia, because they are relevant to treatment options that might be considered (eg assessment of surgical risk) and because the presence of vascular disease would increase the likelihood of symptoms being due to mesenteric ischaemia.

Angiodysplastic bleeding from the colon is said to be more common in patients with aortic valve stenosis.

Drugs
Ask particularly about the use of aspirin, NSAIDs and warfarin.

Family history
The scenario states that this patient's mother had bowel cancer: try to elicit exactly what the problem was. A family history of colorectal carcinoma or colonic polyps strengthens the argument for thorough investigation, particularly in a younger patient, although in this man's case there is no debate: he has caecal carcinoma until proved otherwise. A family history of inflammatory bowel disease might also be relevant, and remember that the rare condition of hereditary haemorrhagic telangiectasia is an autosomal dominant disorder.

Common causes of rectal bleeding

- Haemorrhoids: may have perianal symptoms; do not cause change in bowel habit.
- Colorectal carcinoma: may have change in bowel habit and weight loss; family history is important.
- Diverticular disease: history of chronic constipation and left iliac fossa pain.

Plan for investigation and management
After explaining to the patient that under normal clinical circumstances

you would examine him you would plan as follows.

Routine blood and radiological tests

- FBC: microcytic anaemia suggests chronic blood loss, a raised platelet count inflammation or brisk bleeding.

- Electrolytes, renal and liver function tests: abnormality may be an early indicator of metastatic colorectal neoplasia or suggestive of significant liver disease and therefore of rectal varices; hypoalbuminaemia may be due to protein loss from the gut and/or chronic inflammation.

- Coagulation studies (bleeding diathesis).

- Inflammatory markers: may be substantially raised in diverticulitis and intestinal inflammation.

- Group and save or cross-match blood (if the patient is very anaemic or as a prelude to surgery).

- CXR: look in particular for features of metastatic disease.

Locating the source and cause of rectal bleeding
Frank rectal bleeding can originate anywhere in the gastrointestinal tract, including the upper tract (oesophagus, stomach or duodenum) if haemorrhage is brisk enough. Depending on the circumstances it may therefore be necessary to examine both upper and lower ends of the bowel, but usually only the lower tract needs to be examined. Tests should be selected in the light of the clinical picture, potential benefit, local availability and acceptability to the patient.

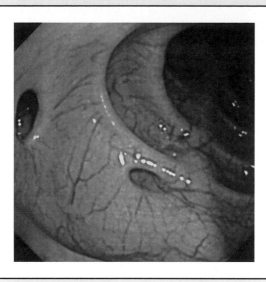

▲**Fig. 5** Two sigmoid diverticula seen at colonoscopy.

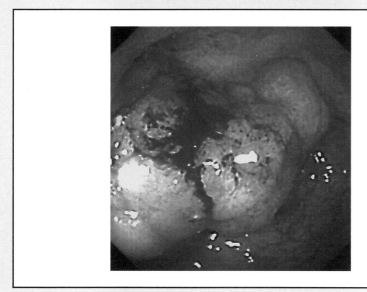

▲**Fig. 6** Colonoscopy showing a colonic carcinoma.

Colonoscopy After proctoscopy/ sigmoidoscopy, this is the preferred investigation in most cases, offering direct visualisation of the entire colon (Figs 5 and 6) and of the terminal ileum, with the ability to take tissue samples and, in some cases, provide therapy, including polypectomy, sclerotherapy, electrocautery, endoclip placement and removal of lesions by endomucosal resection. The procedure is not without risk:

there is a small chance of intestinal perforation (about 1 in 750) and bleeding, which is increased in cases of florid inflammation, obstructing tumours and severe diverticulosis, or when interventions are undertaken.

Barium enema This is generally less reliable than colonoscopy in detecting colonic neoplasia and diverticular disease, cannot diagnose vascular lesions such

as angiodysplasia, and it does not allow the possibility of intervention. It is now rarely used in centres where colonoscopy is readily available.

Mesenteric angiography and red cell scanning Brisk bleeding from a source that cannot be found by other tests can sometimes be identified if the patient can be investigated during the bleeding episode. Angiography has a low yield if employed when the patient is not actively bleeding, but if a source of active bleeding can be identified at angiography then embolisation of the bleeding vessel can often be performed.

Investigation of an abdominal mass

- Radiological imaging: a plain abdominal radiograph may show inflamed loops of bowel appearing as soft-tissue shadowing containing gas. Abdominal ultrasound may reveal thickened bowel loops or an associated abscess. CT scanning is usually the preferred test: it is best able to determine the origin of a mass, and is essential in the full staging of colorectal cancer and lymphoma.

- Laparoscopy/laparotomy: in some patients it may not be possible to fully characterise a mass with non-invasive imaging techniques, in which case direct visualisation and biopsy may be necessary. Surgery may also be needed if there are symptoms suggestive of intestinal obstruction such as nausea or vomiting.

Management
Specific management will depend on the precise diagnosis. Treatment of anaemia by blood transfusion and/or iron supplementation may be required.

TABLE 6 CAUSES OF WEIGHT LOSS IN A YOUNG WOMAN

Type of condition	Cause
Gastrointestinal	Coeliac disease[1] Crohn's disease Pancreatic insufficiency
Endocrine	Diabetes mellitus[1] Thyrotoxicosis[1] Addison's disease
Eating disorder	Deliberate dieting[1] Anorexia nervosa[1]
Chronic infection	Tuberculosis[2]
Malignancy	Haematological

1. Common conditions.
2. Common in high-risk groups.

1.1.5 Weight loss

Letter of referral to gastroenterology clinic

Dear Doctor,

Re: Mrs Sarah Jones, aged 24 years

This young woman has noticed that her clothes are becoming looser-fitting, despite her eating normally, and she is sure that she has lost at least 5 kg in weight, even though she is not on a special diet and has a generally healthy lifestyle. On closer questioning, she has also noticed some diarrhoea recently and feels tired most of the time. I would be most grateful for your assessment.

Yours sincerely,

Introduction

Tiredness is a common and non-specific symptom. Weight is usually fairly constant and loss of 5% or more of the usual body weight must be taken seriously. Although malignancy is an obvious concern, particularly in older patients, in a young woman the diagnoses of malabsorption, thyrotoxicosis, diabetes mellitus and intentional weight loss are more likely (Table 6).

> Diabetes and thyrotoxicosis are very common: diabetes affects 1–2% of the population and thyrotoxicosis affects 1– 2% of women at some time in their lives.

History of the presenting problem

- Weight loss: it is vitally important to actually document this (on the same scales if at all possible). Patient perceptions are sometimes misleading and to embark on a protracted series of investigations for a problem that does not exist is clearly not sensible! If patients have not weighed themselves, ask if clothes/trousers have become looser. Rapid weight loss, particularly in middle-aged or elderly patients, is often associated with malignancy. Ask patients directly if they are trying to lose weight: how does their weight now compare with that 5 and 10 years ago? Have they been on a diet recently, or at any other time?

> Make sure that the patient has actually lost weight before embarking on a hunt for a cause of weight loss.

- Appetite: decreased appetite invariably leads to weight loss and is a feature of many diseases. Weight loss in the context of a good or increased appetite is suggestive of thyrotoxicosis or diabetes mellitus.

- Diarrhoea/steatorrhoea: the latter is a sign of malabsorption and is characterised by loose, oily, bulky, offensive stools that are difficult to flush away. It can be caused by mucosal disease (eg coeliac disease, Crohn's disease) or by pancreatic insufficiency (eg chronic pancreatitis, cystic fibrosis). Remember, however, that diarrhoea does not necessarily imply a primarily gastrointestinal cause of weight loss: it may be a feature of thyrotoxicosis.

- Abdominal pain: should alert to the possibility of Crohn's disease, particularly if located in the right iliac fossa and associated with weight loss. Repeated attacks of central/epigastric pain, especially in the context of high alcohol intake, should raise the possibility of chronic pancreatitis. Pain does not occur in coeliac disease.

Other relevant history

In this young woman it will clearly be very important to enquire if she has had problems with anorexia nervosa or bulimia in the past, also about features that suggest diabetes mellitus (polyuria, polydipsia) or thyrotoxicosis (tremor, agitation, etc.). Family history may be relevant: there is a 10% risk of coeliac disease in the offspring of an affected parent, and diabetes and thyroid disease also have a genetic component.

Unlikely in this woman, but much commoner in an older patient, would be a past history of malignancy. If there is, then onset of weight loss is very suspicious of recurrence or metastatic disease.

Plan for investigation and management

A wide range of conditions can cause tiredness and weight loss, but often the cause is evident after the history and examination such that only a few investigations are necessary. In the absence of an obvious clinical diagnosis the following would be appropriate.

Urine and blood tests

Check urine with dipsticks for glucose, blood and protein. Check FBC, electrolytes, renal/liver/bone function tests, inflammatory markers (erythrocyte sedimentation rate and/or C-reactive protein), glucose, thyroid function tests, 'malabsorption' markers (ferritin, folate, B_{12}), and anti-tissue transglutaminase antibodies (coeliac disease often presents insidiously). Consider short Synacthen test.

> **A raised platelet count may be found with chronic gastrointestinal blood loss, but it is also an 'inflammatory marker' that is often raised in active inflammatory bowel disease, especially Crohn's disease.**

Imaging

- CXR: look for tuberculosis, mediastinal lymphadenopathy, or (very unlikely in this woman, but common in older smokers) bronchial neoplasm or metastatic disease.

- Abdominal ultrasound or (better) CT scanning are non-invasive and may detect inflammatory masses or thickened oedematous loops of small bowel in Crohn's disease, intra-abdominal collections, lymphadenopathy or renal carcinoma.

Other tests

Other investigations may be directed by clinical suspicion or preliminary test results, eg lymph node biopsy, but if there are no clear clinical diagnostic leads and nothing has emerged from the blood tests described, CXR and abdominal imaging, then further investigation is almost certainly not warranted and it is likely that attention can most fruitfully be directed towards psychological causes of tiredness and weight loss, eg eating disorder or depression.

If iron-deficiency anaemia is present, both the upper and lower gastrointestinal tract should be investigated. Barium follow-through or small bowel enema may reveal Crohn's disease. Coeliac disease is confirmed by total or subtotal villous atrophy on duodenal biopsies (Fig. 7).

> ⚠ **Do not forget that the radiological appearances of intestinal tuberculosis may look identical to Crohn's disease, so keep a high index of suspicion, particularly in Asian patients.**

Management

Management will be dictated by the specific diagnosis made.

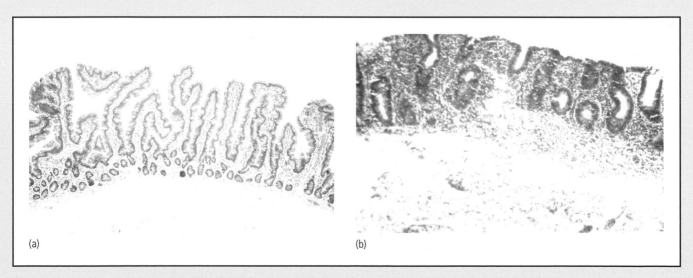

(a)   (b)

▲ **Fig. 7** Coeliac disease: **(a)** histologically normal small bowel with normal villi contrasts with **(b)** total villous atrophy of coeliac disease.

1.1.6 Chronic abdominal pain

Letter of referral to gastroenterology outpatient clinic

Dear Doctor,

Re: Mr Geoffrey Archer, aged 67 years

This man, who does not readily seek medical attention, came to the surgery recently complaining of a 6-month history of crampy epigastric pain and one stone weight loss. He has no significant change in bowel habit but has a history of ischaemic heart disease, hypertension and peripheral vascular disease. Your input into his further investigation and management would be greatly appreciated.

Yours sincerely,

Introduction

The differential diagnosis of chronic abdominal pain is shown in Table 7. In this man there must clearly be concern over the possibility of a malignant cause, but his cardiovascular risk factors make mesenteric ischaemia a possibility. Crohn's disease can present with abdominal pain and weight loss, but the lack of bowel symptoms,

assuming that these have not been missed by the referring doctor, makes this diagnosis less likely.

History of the presenting problem

Related to the pain

- Nature of the pain: is it constant, intermittent or colicky? Colicky pain is characteristic of luminal obstruction (intestinal, biliary or ureteric). Pain that is ever-present is unusual, but should raise the suspicion of malignant disease with local infiltration into neighbouring structures.

- Localisation of pain: gastric pain typically localises to the epigastrium, small bowel pain to the umbilicus and large bowel pain to the iliac fossae; pancreatic pain typically radiates through to the back.

> ⚠ Visceral pain is notoriously difficult to localise: do not be misled as to the site of a problem purely because of the location of the pain.

- Exacerbating or relieving factors: gastric ulcers, mesenteric ischaemia, biliary colic and intestinal obstruction are typically made worse by eating, with biliary colic particularly associated with fatty foods. Duodenal ulcers often

improve after eating. Chronic pancreatitis is worsened by alcohol ingestion.

- Pain at night: nocturnal pain is typically associated with significant pathology and should not be attributed to functional disease (eg irritable bowel syndrome) without thorough investigation to exclude other causes.

Other symptoms

- Weight loss: this man has lost a stone in weight and, as with nocturnal pain, weight loss should raise thoughts of significant pathology and must not be dismissed lightly.

> ⚠ Weight loss does not necessarily indicate malignant disease: it may feature in any condition where eating provokes pain.

- Vomiting: many causes of chronic abdominal pain may be associated with vomiting, but particular thought should be given to peptic ulcer disease and gastric malignancy causing gastric outlet obstruction and intestinal obstruction.

- Change in bowel habit: may be seen in Crohn's disease, irritable bowel syndrome, diverticular disease and colonic malignancy. Chronic pancreatitis may be associated with diarrhoea due to exocrine pancreatic insufficiency.

- Changes suggesting biliary disease: dark urine and/or pale stools.

Other relevant history

A history of previous surgery may suggest adhesions and obstruction. Have there been any previous

TABLE 7 DIFFERENTIAL DIAGNOSIS OF CHRONIC ABDOMINAL PAIN		
Common	**Uncommon**	**Rare**
Peptic ulcer disease	Mesenteric ischaemia	Addison's disease
Gastric carcinoma	Crohn's disease	C1-esterase deficiency
Biliary colic	Subacute bowel obstruction	
Chronic pancreatitis	(adhesions, luminal stricture,	
Pancreatic carcinoma	herniae)	
Diverticular disease		
Irritable bowel syndrome		

episodes of pain, or of problems that might support a diagnosis of Crohn's, eg mouth ulcers, perianal lesions?

Like all arterial diseases, mesenteric ischaemia is associated with hypertension, other atherosclerotic diseases (eg ischaemic heart disease, peripheral vascular disease – both suffered by this man – and stroke), smoking, diabetes and hypercholesterolaemia.

A history of alcohol abuse would raise the possibility of chronic pancreatitis, and a careful drug history is essential: is the patient taking aspirin, NSAIDs or other ulcerogenic drugs?

Plan for investigation and management

Routine blood and radiological tests

- FBC: iron-deficiency anaemia would raise the possibility of upper gastrointestinal blood loss, which in this man with epigastric pain would be most likely due to peptic ulcer disease or gastric malignancy; a raised platelet count can be seen with gastrointestinal blood loss but is also an indicator of inflammation (eg Crohn's disease).

- Electrolytes and renal function tests: in the absence of vomiting or unrelated disease these are likely to be normal; the combination of hyperkalaemia, hyponatraemia and mildly raised urea would raise the very remote possibility of Addison's disease.

- Deranged liver function tests (particularly bilirubin, alkaline phosphatase and γ-glutamyl transaminase) might suggest biliary pathology.

- CXR: particularly for features of metastatic disease.

Amylase is usually normal in chronic pancreatitis.

Endoscopy

In this man, where the epigastric location of pain and presence of weight loss indicates that peptic ulceration or gastric malignancy are the most likely diagnoses, upper gastrointestinal endoscopy is the investigation of choice. In contrast, alteration in bowel habit associated with abdominal pain and weight loss should prompt you to consider colonoscopy.

Radiological tests

- Plain abdominal radiograph and ultrasound scan: there is a limited role for plain radiographs unless you suspect an acute obstructive or ischaemic episode. Pancreatic calcification may be seen in chronic pancreatitis. Ultrasonography may demonstrate gallstones, biliary dilatation, liver metastases or a pancreatic mass.

Gallstones are a common finding, and unless there is corroborative evidence that they might be causing problems (eg abnormal liver function tests, thick-walled gallbladder) they may well be an incidental finding.

- Barium studies: small bowel studies may show strictures in Crohn's disease that are difficult to diagnose in any other way.

- CT and MRI: abdominal CT may show pancreatic masses, pancreatic duct irregularity or calcification (chronic pancreatitis) and can be used to stage gastric or other malignancies and (with newer machines) mesenteric vessel disease. MRI can be used to investigate biliary dilatation (magnetic resonance cholangiopancreatography) or suspected mesenteric ischaemia (magnetic resonance angiography).

CT and MRI are not first-line techniques for the investigation of abdominal pain and will usually be indicated to clarify or stage abnormalities found on ultrasound or endoscopy or, if these have been normal, to further investigate a patient where the index of suspicion is high that there is still an underlying significant pathology.

- Angiography: this remains the investigation of choice for confirming mesenteric ischaemia and also offers the possibility of therapeutic intervention (angioplasty).

Significant mesenteric ischaemia is unlikely unless at least two of the major intestinal arteries are involved, eg coeliac plexus and superior mesenteric artery.

Management

Management will be dictated by the specific diagnosis made.

1.1.7 Abnormal liver function tests

Letter of referral to hepatology outpatient clinic

Dear Doctor,

Re: Mrs Kate Beaumont, aged 50 years

Thank you for seeing this woman who has recently been diagnosed as having diabetes. She has a history of long-standing obesity and more recently of high cholesterol (6.5 mmol/L). Prior to starting her on simvastatin I noted slightly deranged liver function tests [alanine transaminase 85 U/L (normal range 5–40), γ-glutamyltransferase 150 U/L (normal range 7–35)], which have remained abnormal on repeat testing. Physical examination is unrevealing. I would value your opinion as to the cause of these abnormalities.

Yours sincerely,

TABLE 8 LIVER FUNCTION TESTS AND THEIR SIGNIFICANCE

Blood test	Significance of elevated level
Transaminases	Raised serum ALT and AST usually signify hepatocellular damage, but consider other source of AST (heart and skeletal muscle, kidney, red cells) Extreme elevations of AST and ALT occur mainly with drug toxicity, acute viral hepatitis and ischaemic damage to the liver Moderate elevations of AST and ALT are seen in alcohol-related, autoimmune, chronic viral, and other acute and chronic liver disease
Alkaline phosphatase and GGT	These 'biliary' enzymes usually indicate cholestatic liver disease or biliary tract disease GGT levels are disproportionately raised in alcohol-related liver disease, or where an enzyme-inducing drug such as phenytoin or phenobarbital is used Segmental non-obstructive damage to the biliary tree, as in metastatic or infiltrative disease, often produces elevated biliary enzymes, mildly elevated transaminases and normal serum bilirubin Alkaline phosphatase can arise from liver, bone and intestine: determination of isoenzymes can be used to distinguish between these sources
Bilirubin	Where hyperbilirubinaemia is due to excess haem breakdown serum bilirubin is predominantly unconjugated. Unconjugated bilirubinaemia also occurs with inherited disorders of bilirubin conjugation (Gilbert's and Crigler–Najjar syndromes) Conjugated bilirubinaemia can occur with any form of liver damage that interferes with hepatocyte function (intrahepatic cholestasis), but in chronic liver disease is typically a late feature and usually signifies hepatic decompensation Primary diseases of bile canaliculi, ducts and the gallbladder and large bile ducts (PBC, PSC, stones) produce hyperbilirubinaemia and elevated biliary enzymes
Albumin	Albumin is produced in the liver and synthesis declines with worsening liver function. As the half-life of serum albumin is about 30 days, it is days before changes in synthesis are detectable
Prothrombin time	This is a sensitive test of hepatic synthetic capacity as the liver is responsible for the synthesis of factors II (prothrombin), V, VII and IX. The prothrombin time responds rapidly to changes in hepatic synthesis as the serum half-life of clotting factors is of the order of hours

ALT, alanine transaminase; AST, aspartate transaminase; GGT, γ-glutamyltransferase; PBC, primary biliary cirrhosis; PSC, primary sclerosing cholangitis.

Introduction

Reduced liver function is hard to detect clinically, except when the liver is severely impaired. The liver can be markedly damaged without any overt clinical manifestation. The standard liver function tests can provide early warning of potentially serious pathology (Table 8), but significant liver disease, including cirrhosis, can be present with normal liver enzymes. The detection of liver disease relies on the combination of careful clinical assessment, a variety of blood tests, radiological investigations, and often on histological examination of a liver biopsy.

> ⚠️ Significant liver damage, including cirrhosis, may exist with little or no change in serum liver enzyme levels.

Interpretation of liver function tests

- A normal GGT essentially excludes the liver as the source of a raised alkaline phosphatase.
- Reduced serum albumin is part of the acute-phase response, hence levels may be reduced in severe infection even if hepatic function is otherwise normal.

- Prolongation of the prothrombin time may not be due to hepatic synthetic dysfunction: it can be prolonged by vitamin K deficiency resulting from prolonged cholestasis and malabsorption of fat-soluble vitamins.

History of the presenting problem

It is very common for minor abnormalities in liver function to be uncovered by routine screening, particularly prior to initiation of new drugs. Many patients will have no specific symptoms, but ask about general malaise, tiredness, weight loss or gain, loss of libido and sexual potency (in men), and right hypochondrial pain or discomfort.

Other relevant history

In enquiring about relevant history bear in mind the commoner causes of liver enzyme abnormalities [fatty liver (steatosis), alcohol, hepatitis C] and the well-described risk factors for liver disease (previous blood transfusion, previous intravenous drug abuse, diabetes, medication use). Although the history-taking station of PACES is not primarily designed to test communication skills, some of the matters that need to be discussed are potentially sensitive and the examiners (and patients in routine clinical practice) will not be impressed if they are handled in a brutal manner.

This woman has diabetes mellitus, obesity and hyperlipidaemia, which are all associated with hepatic steatosis, but in addition to these important risk factors there may be other reasons why the woman may have abnormal liver function tests. Ask about the following.

- Previous liver disease or jaundice: has the woman had any problem with her liver or with jaundice before? Chronic viral hepatitis

may follow a poorly remembered episode of jaundice, and recurrent episodes of jaundice may signify cholelithiasis. If the only abnormality is mild hyperbilirubinaemia, consider Gilbert's syndrome.

- Alcohol: the most common cause of liver disease in the Western world. Even moderate intake may cause liver damage in susceptible individuals. Be aware of a tendency to minimise drinking when the patient perceives it as morally or socially awkward to be accurate.

- Drugs and medications: prescription drugs, oral contraceptive pill, over-the-counter medications, herbal remedies, traditional medications and recreational drugs should all be considered. Also ask about surgery: recent exposure to anaesthetic agents may have provoked hepatitis, and gastrointestinal surgery for obesity may provoke a steatohepatitis.

- Disease associations: diseases such as primary biliary cirrhosis, primary sclerosing cholangitis and other autoimmune liver diseases are not infrequently associated with other conditions. Ask about coeliac disease, inflammatory bowel disease, thyroid disease, and autoimmune rheumatic disorders (eg scleroderma, Sjögrens syndrome, Raynaud's disease).

- Multisystem disorders: sarcoidosis and various vasculitides can all involve the liver, as may lymphoma and other neoplastic diseases, and infections such as tuberculosis.

- Infections: enquire about travel to or residence in areas endemic for hydatid disease, amoebiasis, schistosomiasis and liver flukes. A patient may not regard it as relevant that he or she lived

in India for 20 years, and the surrogate in PACES may be told not to mention it unless asked directly.

- Family history: ask particularly about a family history of liver disease, inflammatory bowel disease, coeliac disease, hyperlipidaemia and diabetes mellitus (which this woman has). Each of these can be familial and associated with liver abnormalities.

Exceedingly unlikely in a patient of this age, but in a younger patient with unexplained liver disease it is important to consider Wilson's disease and take a neurological/psychiatric history. About 40% of patients with this condition present with liver disease, but in others the first symptoms are either neurological or psychiatric or both, and include tremor, rigidity, drooling, difficulty with speech, abrupt personality change, grossly inappropriate behaviour and an inexplicable deterioration in school work, neurosis or psychosis.

Relevant in a younger woman might be pregnancy, which is associated with a number of hepatic disorders, including cholestasis of pregnancy, HELLP syndrome (*h*aemolysis, *e*levated *l*iver enzyme levels and a *lo*w *p*latelet count) and acute fatty liver of pregnancy.

Plan for investigation and management

After explaining to the patient that under normal clinical circumstances you would examine her to confirm her GP's findings, you would plan as follows.

Blood tests

There are a large number of causes of abnormal liver function tests. The commonest causes of chronic liver disease should always be looked for, including hepatitis B and C, haemochromatosis and autoimmune liver disease, with others depending on clinical suspicion if the diagnosis remains elusive (Table 9).

Imaging

The first-line imaging test should be an abdominal ultrasound scan to look at the liver (is it large, are there abnormal areas, does it look fatty, are its blood vessels normal?), the gallbladder (is there evidence of gallstones?) and spleen (is it large?).

Liver biopsy

Sometimes the information from blood tests and ultrasound examination is not enough to make a confident diagnosis, or the degree of liver damage needs to be more thoroughly assessed in order to stage disease, assess prognosis and guide therapy, in which case a liver biopsy may be indicated (Fig. 8).

Management

Management will be dictated by the specific diagnosis made.

Non-alcoholic fatty liver disease

Non-alcoholic fatty liver disease (NAFLD) is probably the most common liver disease in the developed world. It consists of two stages, fatty liver and non-alcoholic steatohepatitis (NASH), and a liver biopsy is needed to distinguish between them. A fatty liver is generally considered a benign and reversible condition characterised by fat deposits in hepatocytes. NASH describes the progression of fat deposition to inflammation or so-called steatohepatitis, which can lead to fibrosis, cirrhosis and the associated risks of end-stage liver disease (portal hypertension, hepatocellular carcinoma).

The combination of obesity, hyperinsulinaemia, insulin resistance, diabetes, hypertriglyceridaemia and hypertension is known as the metabolic syndrome. NAFLD appears to be the liver component of this syndrome. Treatment of patients with NAFLD is still typically focused on the management of associated conditions such as obesity, diabetes mellitus, hyperlipidaemia and discontinuation of hepatotoxic

---

TABLE 9 DIAGNOSTIC BLOOD TESTS FOR CHRONIC LIVER DISEASE

Alcohol-induced liver disease	May be a raised IgA level, relatively higher AST than ALT, and disproportionately raised GGT
Fatty liver, hepatic steatosis and non-alcoholic steatohepatitis	Associated with diabetes mellitus, so check fasting glucose/glucose tolerance test in patient without known diabetes
Chronic viral hepatitis[1]	HBsAg is the correct screening test; if positive, test for HBeAg, HBV DNA. Note that antibodies to hepatitis B antigens may reflect previous infection or immunisation Anti-HCV antibody is the correct screening test; if positive, test for HCV RNA
Genetic haemochromatosis	Raised serum iron, transferrin saturation and ferritin levels Genetic testing for the common *HFE* mutation may be helpful (positive in 95% of affected individuals)
Autoimmune liver disease	Raised IgG levels, positive autoantibodies (anti-nuclear, anti-smooth muscle, anti-liver and kidney microsomal antigens)
Primary biliary cirrhosis	Positive anti-mitochondrial antibody
α_1-Antitrypsin deficiency	Reduced circulating α_1-antitrypsin, mutant form of protein on electrophoresis
Wilson's disease	Raised serum copper, lowered serum caeruloplasmin level (and increased urinary copper excretion basally and after oral penicillamine challenge)

1. Note that in some cases acute viral hepatitis can be subclinical, so check IgM to hepatitis A, E or B antigens if there is possible exposure.
ALT, alanine transaminase; AST, asparate transaminase; GGT, γ-glutamyltransferase; HBsAg, hepatitis B surface antigen; HBeAg, hepatitis B envelope antigen; HBV, hepatitis B virus; HCV, hepatitis C virus.

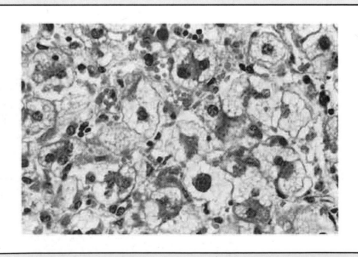

▲**Fig. 8** Microscopic appearance of hepatic steatosis (fatty liver). Fat droplets are seen filling most of the hepatocytes, with the nuclei in the centres of the cells.

drugs known to produce NAFLD (steroids, amiodarone, tamoxifen, methotrexate). There are no specific therapies.

The use of liver biopsy in diagnosing steatohepatitis is still controversial but clinical indicators predicting the diagnosis of the steatohepatitic subset include BMI >30, being diabetic and age over 45 years.

1.1.8 Abdominal swelling

Letter of referral to gastroenterology outpatient clinic

Dear Doctor,

Re: Mrs Bhavani Patel, aged 60 years

This woman came to see me today complaining of increasing abdominal distension. She has no very significant past medical history but has been seen intermittently over the past 3 years with complaints of lethargy and more recently has had difficulty sleeping due to itching. I am grateful for your assessment and advice.

Yours sincerely,

Introduction

It is unusual for abdominal swelling to be an isolated problem: there will often be additional symptoms or an easily identifiable associated history. The most important diagnostic consideration is ascites, the differential diagnosis of which and of other causes of abdominal swelling is given in Table 10.

History of the presenting problem

The following features need to be determined: duration of the swelling, and the presence of associated symptoms such as pain, vomiting, constipation, weight loss or jaundice.

- Duration: intestinal obstruction, paralytic ileus and volvulus typically develop rapidly. Most cases of ascites develop over days to weeks. Fat, faeces, fetal tissue and tumours accumulate over months. Fluctuation in the distention may suggest bloating associated with irritable bowel syndrome.

- Pain: the presence of discomfort due to distension with ascites is common, but constant pain may indicate inflammation or malignancy. A sudden severe pain associated with the development of jaundice would suggest hepatic vein thrombosis (Budd–Chiari syndrome). Colicky pain may suggest intestinal disease, particularly obstruction, and the association of pain with ingestion of food (particularly high fibre) would further support this diagnosis. Pain radiating to the back is typical of pancreatitis, a rare but important cause of ascites.

- Vomiting: the presence of vomiting suggests intestinal obstruction, particularly if in large volume, faeculent, projectile or persistent.

- Change in bowel habit: ask about constipation, particularly in the elderly, mentally ill or those in residential or nursing homes. Ileus or intestinal obstruction results in diminished bowel movements or even total constipation (absence of passage of faeces or flatus). In some instances, particularly in the presence of a stoma, the patient may notice a slowing of bowel function followed by explosive defecation in the instance of subacute obstruction.

- Weight loss: the accumulation of fluid in ascites will obviously lead to weight gain, but if the patient has lost weight or muscle bulk

TABLE 10 DIFFERENTIAL DIAGNOSIS OF ASCITES/ABDOMINAL SWELLING			
Common	**Uncommon**	**Rare**	**Non-ascitic causes of abdominal swelling**
Decompensated chronic liver disease	Acute liver failure (ascites is relatively uncommon at the	Peritoneal tuberculosis	Chronic constipation
Alcoholic hepatitis	time of presentation)	Right-sided heart failure/ constrictive pericarditis	Gaseous distension
	Budd–Chiari syndrome (acute hepatic vein occlusion)	Acute pancreatitis	Acute bowel obstruction/ paralytic ileus
	Peritoneal carcinomatosis	Nephrotic syndrome	Massive organomegaly
	Ovarian carcinoma	Myxoedema	Obesity
			Pregnancy

then this may indicate an underlying malignant process. Patients with advanced alcoholic liver disease are also likely to have lost significant body mass.

> 🔑 The presence of jaundice suggests a hepatic cause for ascites, but remember that the absence of jaundice does not exclude it.

- Other symptoms suggesting liver disease: fatigue and pruritis are often presenting features of chronic liver disease (and present in this scenario).

Other relevant history

Given that ascites related to chronic liver disease is the most likely diagnosis, it is essential to probe tactfully for evidence that the patient may have, or may be at risk of, chronic liver disease. After preliminary questions such as 'Have you ever had jaundice or liver disease in the past?' it will be necessary to explore a careful alcohol history and explore risk factors for hepatitis C (and B), including blood transfusion (pre-1992 and abroad), intravenous drug use and high-risk sexual behaviour.

Ask about other diseases associated with liver disease: inflammatory bowel disease (especially ulcerative colitis) is associated with primary sclerosing cholangitis; coeliac disease and other autoimmune diseases are associated with primary biliary cirrhosis. A family history of liver disease should lead to consideration of haemochromatosis (and other rare conditions).

Clearly not relevant in this case, but a menstrual history should be taken from a younger woman, looking both for unexpected pregnancy and gynaecological malignancy;

postmenopausal bleeding could clearly be significant in this case.

Plan for investigation and management

> 🔑 Many patients associate the term 'cirrhosis' with alcohol: it is important to state that it represents scarring and can have many causes, which the tests will help to determine.

Blood tests

Routine blood tests will include the following.

- FBC: hypersplenism (low platelet count, pancytopenia), alcoholic aetiology (raised mean corpuscular volume).

- Electrolytes, urea and creatinine.

- Transaminases, alkaline phosphatase and γ-glutamyltransferase (see Section 1.1.7).

> ⚠️ Beware of the patient with alcoholic liver disease and urea or creatinine at the upper limit of normal: very low levels are expected and a 'normal' value almost certainly indicates significant renal impairment.

Assessment of liver function

The best indicators of liver function are prothrombin time, serum albumin and bilirubin: it would be highly unlikely that there is a hepatic cause for ascites if these are all normal.

Assessment directed to the cause of liver disease

A 'non-invasive liver screen' would be indicated if there were abnormalities of transaminases, alkaline phosphatase or

γ-glutamyltransferase. In brief this would include the following.

- Viral serology: hepatitis B and C.

- Immunology: autoantibodies including anti-nuclear antigen (ANA), anti-mitochondrial antibody (AMA), smooth muscle antibody (SMA) and immunoglobulin levels.

- Serum ferritin, iron and iron-binding studies: a ferritin level persistently greater than 1000 µg/L is highly suggestive of haemochromatosis and should prompt genetic testing for the *HFE* gene (abnormal in ~95% of cases).

- α_1-Antitrypsin level.

- Copper evaluation (Wilson's disease).

- Alpha-fetoprotein (AFP): in patients with known liver disease who decompensate (become jaundiced, encephalopathic or develop ascites) unexpectedly consider hepatocellular carcinoma.

> 🔑 Ferritin levels are often elevated in liver disease irrespective of causation.

> ⚠️ AFP may be normal in 10–20% of cases of hepatocellular cancer.

Imaging

- Plain abdominal radiograph: if bowel obstruction or ileus is suspected.

- Abdominal ultrasound: this may confirm the diagnosis of ascites, especially if the amount of free fluid is small. It will also provide evidence on the nature of the liver (size, texture) and the presence of focal lesions. The flow through the portal vein should be requested (retrograde flow is usually indicative of portal hypertension and cirrhosis and will also determine the presence or absence of thrombus here, which may have implications for future management since it may preclude shunt placement or transplantation). Splenomegaly is suggestive of portal hypertension.

- CT/MRI: the suspicion of hepatocellular carcinoma requires imaging by either MRI or triphasic CT scanning and referral to the relevant hepatobiliary specialist. Other causes of ascites may be revealed, including ovarian masses and peritoneal thickening due to malignant infiltration.

Ascitic aspiration

Send for leucocytes, microscopy and culture, albumin, amylase and cytology. Spontaneous bacterial peritonitis (SBP) is a serious complication of ascites associated with chronic liver disease and is diagnosed by a leucocyte count >250 cells/mL in the ascitic fluid. Compare ascitic albumin concentration with serum albumin concentration: a gradient >11 g/L suggests portal hypertension; a gradient <11 g/L suggests an exudative cause (neoplastic, infective or pancreatitis).

Liver biopsy

> ⚠️ Percutaneous liver biopsy should *not* be performed in the presence of ascites. It is questionable whether any approach to liver biopsy is safe, but the best would be to drain the ascites and proceed to transjugular biopsy if a tissue diagnosis is needed.

Management

In most patients the presence of ascites should prompt admission for investigation and treatment.

Specific treatment Any specific underlying cause of chronic liver disease should be treated if possible, including abstinence in alcoholic liver disease, steroids in autoimmune hepatitis and venesection in haemochromatosis.

> 🔑 Decompensated cirrhosis may improve if the 'insult' (eg alcohol) is removed.

Antibiotic therapy with a quinolone or a third-generation cephalosporin should be initiated immediately in the presence of SBP. A patient with chronic liver disease and a history of previous SBP or a low ascites protein level (<10 g/L) should be treated with prophylactic antibiotics to avoid the condition.

> ⚠️ Cultures in spontaneous bacterial peritonitis are often negative and waiting for them should not delay treatment.

Symptomatic management of ascites The following therapies may be appropriate.

- Diuretics: most ascites should be treated initially with a diuretic. Begin with spironolactone, and note that here is usually a delay of 2–3 days between introduction of the drug and initial effect. Careful use of furosemide may be required but can precipitate dramatic hyponatraemia.

> ⚠️ Significant renal impairment as well as hyperkalaemia can be induced by diuretics: progress should be monitored by daily weights (reduce diuretics if weight loss >1 kg/day) and fastidious renal monitoring.

- Fluid and salt restriction: restriction of fluid intake to 1–1.5 L/day is often recommended, as is salt restriction, but patients often fail to comply.

- Paracentesis: in the distressed patient or those who fail to respond to diuretics therapeutic paracentesis is required. Recurrent reaccumulation of ascites may be an indication for referral for consideration of transplantation or portosystemic shunting (eg transjugular intrahepatic portosystemic shunt).

Further discussion

Varices

Any patient with suspected cirrhosis or portal hypertension should be screened for oesophageal varices.

Albumin infusion

The benefits of human albumin solution in patients with ascites and renal dysfunction, or in those undergoing paracentesis, are controversial and poorly understood. In simplistic terms it acts as a small-volume plasma expander, improving renal perfusion and function in hepatorenal syndrome (2 units/day) and prevents circulatory collapse and hepatorenal syndrome after large-volume paracentesis. For paracentesis, 100 mL of 20% human albumin solution per 2–3 L drained is usually administered.

1.2 Clinical examination

1.2.1 Inflammatory bowel disease

General features

In routine clinical practice the first concern is always whether the patient is well, unwell or extremely unwell, but patients who are acutely unwell are not likely to appear in a PACES examination. Important issues to comment on before proceeding to examination of the abdomen itself include the following.

- Nutritional status: does the patient look well-nourished? If given the opportunity to ask, say that you would like to know his weight/height/BMI.

- Hands: clubbing, leuconychia.

- Eyes: anaemia is a frequent complication of Crohn's disease and iritis an association.

- Mouth: aphthous ulceration.

- Legs: erythema nodosum; peripheral oedema due to hypoproteinaemia.

- Features of chronic liver disease (see Section 1.2.2): primary sclerosing cholangitis (PSC) may complicate ulcerative colitis or Crohn's disease.

Abdominal examination

External examination of the abdomen may be unremarkable, but look and palpate carefully for the following.

- Scars: about 80% of patients with Crohn's disease and 20% of those with ulcerative colitis undergo abdominal surgery over a lifetime.

- Palpable bowel: a thickened fibrosed segment of sigmoid colon may be felt in ulcerative colitis; Crohn's disease (also ileocaecal tuberculosis) may cause an ill-defined tender mass in the right iliac fossa.

Rectal examination

This is mandatory in clinical practice and should be commented on, although not performed, in the setting of the PACES examination. Features to look for would include signs of:

- excoriation at the anal verge (may result from excess secretions);

- ulceration, fissuring and scarring (signs of anorectal involvement);

- blood and pus (indicative of active proctitis/colitis).

Further discussion

Abdominal examination may be completely normal in cases of inflammatory bowel disease, but it is likely that at least some features of the general or specific examination will be abnormal in a patient appearing in PACES (although a patient with no abnormal physical signs can be included).

If you could feel a mass, what is the differential diagnosis of the findings?

Could colorectal neoplasia mimic inflammatory bowel disease? As cancer can complicate long-standing active colitis, this is an important practical question and the presence of a mass would require investigation with CT and/or colonoscopy.

If this man presented with bloody diarrhoea, how would you manage him?

See Sections 1.1.3 and 1.4.2.

1.2.2 Chronic liver disease

General features

The only common cause of haematemesis associated with abnormal physical signs is chronic liver disease and the statement that the patient had a 'brisk, painless, large-volume haematemesis' is clearly a pointer to varices. In routine practice your first concern would be to assess the state of the circulation, but patients who are actively bleeding will not (or should not) appear in PACES. What evidence of chronic liver disease might be apparent from the end of the bed?

- General appearance: is the patient cachectic? If given the opportunity to ask, say that you would like to know his weight/height/BMI. Gynaecomastia, loss of secondary sexual hair (in men); tanned appearance (consider haemochromatosis).

- Skin: jaundice, spider naevi, bruising, scratch marks; tattoos, signs of intravenous drug abuse (risk factors for hepatitis B and C).

- Hands: liver flap, clubbing, leuconychia, palmar erythema, Dupuytren's contracture.

- Eyes: jaundice, anaemia.

- Mouth: angular cheilosis, poor dentition.

- Abdomen: may be obviously distended.

- Legs: 'tissue paper' skin; peripheral oedema due to hypoproteinaemia.

Also look for the following.

- Cushingoid features: suggest long-term steroid treatment.

- Pigmentation: consider haemochromatosis ('bronze diabetes').

- Telangiectasiae on the face, lips and within the mouth: these would indicate that the patient almost certainly has hereditary haemorrhagic telangiectasiae, a rare autosomal dominant condition associated with gastrointestinal bleeding that appears in medical examinations, including PACES, with inordinate frequency.

Abdominal examination

Comment on the presence or absence of the following.

- Distension.

- Prominent anterior abdominal wall veins with flow away from the umbilicus ('caput medusa').

- Hepatomegaly: but remember that most causes of chronic liver disease are associated with a shrunken liver. Listen for a bruit.

- Splenomegaly: the key physical sign indicating the presence of portal hypertension in a patient with chronic liver disease, although the absence of splenomegaly does not mean that portal hypertension can be excluded.

- Ascites: test for shifting dullness.

Rectal examination for the formal assessment of melaena remains essential in routine clinical practice, and a comment to this effect would be appropriate in PACES.

TABLE 11 CAUSES OF CHRONIC LIVER DISEASE

Frequency	Condition
Common	Alcoholic liver disease Chronic viral hepatitis: hepatitis C or hepatitis B Non-alcoholic steatohepatitis
Less common	Autoimmune liver diseases: primary biliary cirrhosis, autoimmune hepatitis, primary sclerosing cholangitis Cryptogenic or idiopathic (represents probably <20% of cases now)
Rare	Metabolic and genetic liver diseases: α_1-antitrypsin deficiency, haemochromatosis, Wilson's disease Infiltrative liver disease: sarcoidosis, amyloidosis Miscellaneous: secondary biliary cirrhosis, prolonged total parenteral nutrition, cystic fibrosis, chronic heart failure

Further discussion

What are the common causes of chronic liver disease?
See Table 11.

How would you investigate if you suspected chronic liver disease?
See Section 1.1.7.

How would you manage the patient if presenting with a further gastrointestinal bleed?
See Section 1.4.3.

In what diseases can patients have variceal haemorrhage but not chronic liver disease?
Portal hypertension can be divided into prehepatic, hepatic and posthepatic types (Table 12).

Thus it is possible to have normal liver function and still bleed from varices, the commonest causes of this in practice being portal and splenic vein thrombosis.

1.2.3 Splenomegaly

Instruction

This 35-year-old woman has upper abdominal discomfort. Please examine her abdomen.

General features

Look for features of chronic liver disease (as described in Section 1.2.2) and for evidence of haematological disease: pallor/polycythaemia, indwelling

TABLE 12 CAUSES OF PORTAL HYPERTENSION

Prehepatic	Hepatic	Posthepatic
Increased flow (eg arteriovenous fistula, massive splenomegaly) Portal or splenic vein thrombosis (eg pancreatitis, malignancy, sepsis, thrombophilia) Portal vein stenosis (eg post liver transplant)	Presinusoidal (eg primary biliary cirrhosis, schistosomiasis, congenital hepatic fibrosis) Sinusoidal (eg cirrhosis, acute alcoholic hepatitis, fulminant hepatitis) Postsinusoidal (eg veno-occlusive disease)	Hepatic vein outflow obstruction (eg Budd–Chiari syndrome, heart failure, inferior vena cava web)

tunnelled line (for chemotherapy), lymphadenopathy.

Abdominal examination

Observe for scars and obvious swellings before beginning to palpate. After gentle palpation in all quadrants to detect very obvious masses and to see if the patient is tender anywhere, examine for hepatomegaly, splenomegaly and renal enlargement using standard technique. Look for the other features described in Section 1.2.2.

Further discussion

What are the common causes of splenomegaly?
See Table 13.

How would you investigate a patient found to have splenomegaly or hepatosplenomegaly?

- Blood tests: FBC and blood film, routine biochemistry (especially liver and bone profiles), inflammatory markers.

- Radiological investigation: CXR (hilar lymphadenopathy), CT abdomen.

- Other tests: as determined by clinical suspicion, eg bone marrow, screen for causes of chronic liver disease.

1.2.4 Abdominal swelling

> ## Instruction
>
> This man has abdominal swelling. Please examine his abdomen.

General features

In routine clinical practice the first priority would be determine whether the patient was acutely unwell, in which case acute intestinal obstruction would be the immediate concern. Patients with ileus, pseudo-obstruction or constipation are generally less unwell, although they may vomit (look for a sick bowl). Patients with ascites can be moribund (acute hepatitis, Budd–Chiari syndrome), quite

well (chronic diuretic-resistant ascites) or anything in between. Massive organomegaly (hepatomegaly, splenomegaly, hepatosplenomegaly or very large kidneys) can also cause abdominal swelling. In the context of a PACES examination, ascites and organomegaly are much the most likely diagnoses.

From the foot of the bed comment on the following.

- General appearance: is the patient well-nourished? Alcoholic liver disease is often associated with muscle wasting, as is malignant disease, although this would be uncommon in PACES.

- Signs of chronic liver disease: see Section 1.2.2.

- Signs of chronic renal disease: arteriovenous fistulae in the wrist(s) or elbow(s), or signs of previous surgery relating to these; central venous dialysis catheter.

- Signs of haematological disease: petechiae/purpura; indwelling central line for chemotherapy.

Abdominal examination

The specific features of chronic liver disease and hepatosplenomegaly are covered in Sections 1.2.2 and 1.2.3.

- What is the nature of the swelling? Is the abdomen doughy (chronic constipation), gassy (tense, tympanic: ileus, pseudo-obstruction or acute obstruction) or fluid filled (ascites, dialysate), or is the swelling due to organomegaly? In this scenario in PACES ascites is much the most likely diagnosis.

- Is there ascites? Check for shifting dullness; look for dressings, stitches or scars that might indicate recent paracentesis; note if there is umbilical eversion and/or herniation.

TABLE 13 CAUSES OF SPLENOMEGALY

Frequency[1]	Condition
Common	Myeloproliferative diseases (chronic myeloid leukaemia, polycythaemia rubra vera, myelofibrosis) Lymphoproliferative diseases (Hodgkin's disease/non-Hodgkin's lymphoma, chronic lymphoid leukaemia) Portal hypertension
Less common	Chronic infections (eg malaria[2], schistosomiasis[2]) Systemic disease (eg sarcoidosis, amyloidosis, SLE) Thalassaemia major
Rare	Acute infections (eg infectious mononucleosis, bacterial endocarditis, typhoid) Storage diseases (eg Gaucher's, Niemann–Pick) Acute leukaemia Haemolytic anaemia

1. 'Frequency' refers to the context of a PACES examination in the UK.
2. Very common causes in parts of the world where these diseases are endemic.
SLE, systemic lupus erythematosus.

• Is the patient on peritoneal dialysis (Tenckhoff catheter) or does he have a renal transplant ('hockey-stick' scar in right or left iliac fossa with transplant kidney palpable beneath this)? If so, take particular care to palpate bimanually for polycystic kidneys, and note that a large midline abdominal scar or extensive flank incision may indicate that one or both native kidneys have been removed.

If the patient has ascites, then it would be appropriate to look for evidence of right heart failure (is the JVP grossly elevated?) and say that you would like to perform urinalysis to exclude nephrotic syndrome (heavy proteinuria). Also, note if the patient looks hypothyroid, although this would be a very rare cause of ascites indeed.

Further discussion

What is the differential diagnosis of a patient presenting with ascites?
See Table 14.

How would you investigate a patient presenting with ascites?
See Section 1.1.8 and Table 15.

1.3 Communication skills and ethics

1.3.1 A decision about feeding

TABLE 14 CAUSES OF ASCITES

Frequency	Causes
Common	Cirrhosis with portal hypertension
	Malignancy[1]
	Severe congestive cardiac failure
Less common	Budd–Chiari syndrome
	Constrictive pericarditis
	Nephrotic syndrome
Rare	Pancreatic disease
	Hypothyroidism
	Malabsorption (or other cause of hypoalbuminaemia)

1. Rare in PACES.

TABLE 15 DIAGNOSTIC APPROACH TO THE PATIENT WITH ASCITES

Test	Details
Ascitic fluid	Microscopy: malignant cells, infection
	Chemistry: gradient of serum albumin from serum to ascitic fluid of >11 g/L suggests portal hypertension; gradient of <11 g/L suggests an exudative cause (neoplastic, infective)
	Culture: including for tuberculosis
Blood tests	FBC
	Liver function tests: bilirubin, transaminases, alkaline phosphatase, γ-glutamyltransferase, albumin, prothrombin time
Imaging	CXR: looking for evidence of malignancy
	Ultrasound: to confirm ascites and to look at the liver and spleen and (if appropriate) Doppler studies of the portal and hepatic veins

Further investigations will be dictated by clinical suspicion and the results of initial laboratory tests, eg to pursue the cause of chronic liver disease (see Section 1.2.2), possible malignancy (CT scan, biopsy of abnormal tissue) or cardiac dysfunction (ECG, echocardiography).

Scenario

Role: you are a junior doctor working on a medical ward.

Miss Fiona Davies is the daughter of one of your patients. She is concerned about the current condition of her father, Mr Harry Davies, a 72-year-old man with a history of hypertension and mild short-term memory problems who was admitted 2 weeks ago with a stroke that has left him with a marked left-sided weakness and poor swallowing. Over the past week there have been no signs of improvement in his swallowing when assessed by the speech and language therapists. Plans for his long-term care are in progress and early indications are that he will require full care in a nursing home setting.

He has been receiving nutrition via a nasogastric tube, but this has been intermittent as he has not tolerated it well and the tube has become dislodged on several occasions. Plans for his feeding have been discussed and the multidisciplinary team have considered that a percutaneous endoscopic gastrostomy (PEG) would be appropriate. The medical team think that

Mr Davies is able to consent to the procedure. Miss Davies has come to the ward by appointment to discuss long-term feeding issues.

Your task: to explain to Miss Davies what options there are for feeding her father and the recommendation that he has a PEG.

Key issues to explore

Begin by establishing what the daughter's main concerns are. Things that she might want to discuss include different options for maintaining hydration and feeding, her father's capacity to understand and consent to an intervention such as a PEG, and long-term plans for care in the event of his condition deteriorating.

Key points to establish

- That you will listen to any of the daughter's concerns, but that providing artificial hydration and nutrition is a medical intervention and the decision about whether to do so is a medical one, informed by the multidisciplinary team.

- That the view of the medical team is that her father has the capacity to make a decision about his feeding.

- That any decision made will be reviewed if there is any change in her father's condition.

Appropriate responses to likely questions

Daughter: I don't think he'd want to be messed about. Why can't you just keep letting him try to eat and drink?

Doctor: this is something that we have considered. We always prefer a patient to drink and eat normally if they can, but I'm afraid that the stroke has damaged the nerves that control his swallowing. This means that when he tries to eat or drink he coughs and splutters, and some of the food or drink goes down the wrong way and is in danger of landing up in the lungs. If this happens he will get pneumonia, from which he'd be unlikely to recover.

Daughter: but a PEG tube into the stomach sounds horrible. Isn't there anything else that would be better?

Doctor: I understand what you're saying. A PEG tube does sound rather alarming, but it sounds worse than it is. We've already tried feeding him with a tube through the nose into the stomach – a nasogastric tube – and he found that very irritating and kept dislodging it: many people do. A PEG tube obviously doesn't go through the nose, but straight through the abdominal wall and into the stomach, so patients find it much less irritating.

Daughter: how can you be sure that he understands what having a PEG tube means?

Doctor: I agree that it can be difficult to know exactly what a patient understands sometimes. However, we have talked to your father about the reasons for recommending that he has a PEG on several occasions, and we think that he understands the issues: he knows that he needs to have food and drink, he knows that he can't eat and drink normally, and he knows that the tube through the nose is uncomfortable and keeps falling out. We've explained to him how a PEG tube is put in, and the problems that can sometimes arise.

Daughter: so how is a PEG tube put in?

Doctor: a PEG is inserted in the endoscopy department using a special telescope that is passed through the mouth into the stomach. The patient is given a sedative injection if they need one, and local anaesthetic is used in the throat and stomach wall. When the telescope is in the stomach its light can be seen through the skin. A small needle and guidewire are then put through the skin into the stomach from the outside, which the telescope can catch and which is then used to pull the PEG tube into position (Fig. 9).

Daughter: will he need this PEG for the rest of his life?

Doctor: I don't know, but it's possible that he will. Some patients with swallowing difficulties caused by a stroke can improve as time goes on. Sometimes they improve to the point of not needing the PEG any more, in which case it can be removed very simply by pulling it out.

Daughter: what are the risks of putting in a PEG?

Doctor: in most cases the business of putting in a PEG is very straightforward, but you are right in thinking that this isn't always the case. The risks are related to having the telescope inserted into the stomach and to the procedure itself: in a very few cases it isn't possible to put in a PEG; some patients experience bleeding from the stomach afterwards, but this is usually very minor and settles on its own; and sometimes the PEG tube falls out of the stomach into the stomach cavity which can cause irritation. But 18 or 19 out of 20 people have a PEG put in without any problems.

Daughter: will he be able to do things in the day if he is attached to his PEG for feeding?

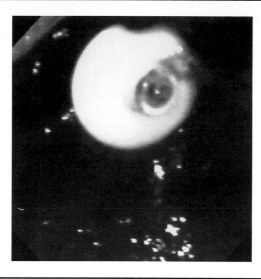

▲**Fig. 9** View of a PEG feeding tube in the stomach at endoscopy.

Doctor: yes, we try to do all the feeding overnight so that the day is freed up for other things such as physiotherapy.

Daughter: will the PEG be obvious?

Doctor: not when it is not being used. When your father is not attached to the feeding bag and tube, the PEG tube lies close to the skin and is not usually visible under clothes.

Daughter: what would happen if we chose not to put in a PEG?

Doctor: if we cannot give him adequate nourishment and hydration, he will deteriorate and would find activities such as physiotherapy more difficult. We think that other methods of trying to give him food and drink will be less effective and have more problems than a PEG.

Further discussion

Any form of artificial feeding is a therapeutic intervention and informed consent from the patient or carers with legal authority must be sought.

The question of artificial nutrition in a patient in a persistent vegetative state was considered by the High Court in 1993, and four principles were established:

- the best interests of the patient is to be the guiding principle;
- artificial nutrition is considered a medical intervention;
- withholding and withdrawing artificial nutrition are equivalent acts;
- it is not unlawful to withhold or withdraw artificial nutrition.

Anorexia nervosa is considered a psychiatric condition and a patient may be detained and treated (eg artificially fed) under the terms of the Mental Health Act.

1.3.2 Limitation of management

Scenario

Role: you are a junior doctor working on a general medical take.

Mrs Agnes Keane, a 93-year-old woman resident in a nursing home, presents with a massive haematemesis on a background of long-standing heart failure and chronic renal failure. She requires full care in the home for all activities of daily living, both because of her heart disease and her advanced dementia. On arrival in the Medical Assessment Unit she is unresponsive, has an unrecordable BP and is pale, with fresh blood around her mouth and melaena stool evident in the bed. An intravenous drip has been put in and resuscitation with colloid commenced by the Emergency Department staff, who ask you to assess her. You contact the on-call medical consultant who decides that Mrs Keane should not undergo further investigation or treatment but should be kept comfortable.

Your task: to explain the situation and management plan to Mrs Keane's daughter.

Key issues to explore

Begin by finding out the daughter's understanding of her mother's condition: although the situation seems clear-cut, it cannot safely be assumed that the daughter will recognise this. Therefore, you need to explore the daughter's expectations of what the outcome is likely to be, and also what she believes her mother would want with regard to treatment and investigation.

Key points to establish

- That Mrs Keane is dying.
- The inappropriateness of aggressive medical interventions

in the context of a patient who is dying.

- That you will listen to the daughter's concerns, but that you will not ask her to make decisions about offering or declining particular treatments, which are medical decisions.

- That doctors are not obliged to provide treatments that they consider to be futile.

Appropriate responses to likely questions

Daughter: why is my mother bleeding from her mouth?

Doctor: I'm afraid that we don't know for certain. The blood is coming from her gut, and it is most likely that she has developed an ulcer in her stomach or the top of her small bowel: this has probably developed over a small blood vessel which is now bleeding.

Daughter: why is my mother unconscious?

Doctor: she has bled so much that her blood pressure has dropped very low. This means that blood is not getting to her brain properly.

Daughter: how are you going to stop the bleeding?

Doctor: there isn't an easy way to do this, and we don't think it would be right to put her through a lot of investigations and treatments that wouldn't do any good and which would cause her distress. The most important thing is that we make sure that she is comfortable.

Daughter: so are you just going to let her bleed to death?

Doctor: I'm sorry, but I'm afraid that your mother is dying. As you know, she has problems with a poor heart, poor kidneys and her mind has gone with dementia, and in the situation

she is in now she would be very unlikely to survive for more than a short while whatever we did. We are going to make sure that she is comfortable: it would be wrong for us to prolong her dying.

Daughter: but I know that you can do telescope tests. Wouldn't it be right to find out what is wrong for sure?

Doctor: at the moment it wouldn't be safe to have a look into your mother's stomach with a telescope. She is unconscious and could not protect her airway, and her blood pressure is too low for the heart to take the strain. If we were to try to do a telescope test we would have to begin by putting her on a breathing machine and giving her a lot of fluid to bring up her blood pressure. Even if we did that it wouldn't be guaranteed that the test could be done safely, or that it would be able to find out what's going on. It really wouldn't be kind or sensible to do this.

Daughter: have you talked to your consultant about this?

Doctor: yes I have, and what I'm explaining to you is what he has asked me to say. If you want to speak to him directly then I can try to arrange this. Would you like me to?

Daughter: how long will it be before she dies?

Doctor: I cannot say for sure, not because I'm hiding anything but because I don't know. She has bled a lot and her blood pressure is very low. She could die very soon – over the next few minutes – or it could be longer if the bleeding slows down, which it can sometimes do.

Daughter: are you sure that she's not in any distress?

Doctor: yes, she isn't responding at all at the moment. She is unconscious and can't feel anything.

But if she did seem to become distressed, if she seemed to be in any pain, then we would give her something to make sure she was comfortable.

1.3.3 Limitation of investigation

Scenario

Role: you are a junior doctor working in a gastroenterology outpatient clinic.

Mr David Chan is a 25-year-old man who has experienced symptoms of irritable bowel syndrome for 8 years and has been extensively investigated previously. He is convinced that his symptoms have worsened considerably and is particularly worried about a recent bout of constipation because he thinks it might indicate cancer. A physical examination is unremarkable and routine tests such as FBC are entirely normal. He wishes to have a colonoscopy, but the consultant who saw him previously said that this was not indicated and declined to perform the investigation.

Your task: to explain to the patient the reasons why the test is not indicated nor on offer, and what the nature of irritable bowel syndrome is.

Key issues to explore

This is clearly going to be a difficult discussion. Begin by asking the patient to explain to you what he thinks is causing his problems, and what his fears and concerns are. Constipation is a common symptom in irritable bowel syndrome (IBS), so is there any particular reason why he is worried about cancer now?

Key points to establish

- You recognise that IBS causes distressing symptoms, but it is benign in the long term, ie it does not lead to excess mortality or predispose to developing other conditions such as colorectal cancer and inflammatory bowel disease.

- Decisions about investigations depend on balancing benefits and risks, and colonoscopy is not without hazards.

- Doctors are not obliged to offer tests or treatments that they do not think are clinically indicated.

Appropriate responses to likely questions

Patient: how can you be sure that I don't have cancer?

Doctor: even if you do every test possible, it cannot be proved that cancer is impossible. But everything we know about you, including the fact that your symptoms have been going on for a long time, that everything is as it should be on examination and that routine blood tests are normal, are reassuring that you do not have a serious disorder such as cancer.

Patient: why don't you just organise a colonoscopy? I'll feel better, and you can get on with your other work.

Doctor: no, this wouldn't be the right thing to do. Deciding about tests or procedures is a matter of balancing benefits and risks, and colonoscopy does carry a small risk of serious complications, such as perforation of the bowel. It wouldn't be right to put you or any patient at risk of this if there wasn't a proper reason for doing the test.

Patient: you're just trying to save money by not doing the test, aren't you?

Doctor: no, that's not the main reason for me saying that we won't do the test. The main reason is because the test stands more chance of doing you harm than doing you good, although I agree that it isn't right to spend healthcare money on something that isn't justified.

Patient: I have a right to have the test, haven't I?

Doctor: no, that's not true. No patient has a right to a test or a treatment that is not clinically indicated. You do have a right to have a second opinion if you want it, and if you'd like me or your GP to recommend someone then we can do, but you can't insist that we do a test that we don't think is justified.

Patient: you think I'm just a whinger, don't you?

Doctor: no, that's not what I've said and it's not what I think. There is no doubt that the symptoms of irritable bowel syndrome exist and can be really severe and worrying; and I and the other doctors in the clinic will help as much as we can to control them. However, we won't do things that we don't think will help.

1.3.4 A patient who does not want to give a history

Scenario

Role: you are a junior doctor working on a general medical ward.

Ms Cathy Evans, a 34-year-old woman who says that she has recently moved to the area and is not registered with a GP, is admitted with episodic severe abdominal pain. At times this seems to be excruciating, such that she rolls around in agony and calls out for pethidine, but

between attacks she seems well and appears unconcerned about her condition. Examination reveals two laparotomy scars, the indications for which are unclear. Routine laboratory tests and plain radiographs are normal. She has been on the ward for 3 days and matters do not seem to be improving. It is the opinion of your consultant that the woman has factitious abdominal pain and that no further investigations should be performed. Ms Evans is unhappy with the lack of investigation since admission and has demanded to see someone to discuss this. Your consultant has asked you to get more information regarding her background history, which Ms Evans has been unwilling to provide.

Your task: to explain to Ms Evans that further details of her medical background are required and that further investigation is not indicated.

Key issues to explore

This is clearly going to be a difficult discussion. Begin by asking the patient to explain to you what she thinks is causing her pain and what she thinks should be done about it. Use comments made by her, which she will almost certainly intend as justification for investigation, as reasons for needing precise details of her past medical history.

Key points to establish

- Reassure her that the progress of her illness and the results of investigation do not indicate serious intra-abdominal pathology.

- Be firm and persistent in requesting specific details: when, which hospital and which doctor, etc? But do not become confrontational.

- Doctors are not obliged to offer tests or treatments that they do not think are clinically indicated.

Appropriate responses to likely questions

Patient: *you haven't found out what's wrong with me yet? Don't I need a CT scan?*

Doctor: you are right that we haven't got to the bottom of things yet, but the tests that we have done have not revealed anything worrying, which is good news. We don't think that a CT scan will add anything useful at this time, but we do need to find out as much as we can about the previous problems you've had in your abdomen, just in case these are relevant to what's happening now.

Patient: *my past isn't relevant, why do I have to tell you about it?*

Doctor: you don't have to tell me anything that you don't want to, but it is very difficult for us to manage you safely without knowing about your past medical history, in particular about the operations that you have had. These details may help us get to the bottom of your current problems and we could miss things if we do not have all the information. Can you remember in which hospital you had them done, and when?

Patient: *what is causing the pain?*

Doctor: we're not sure, but we don't think there is a serious problem in your abdomen. Pain can be caused by a number of things, not all of which can be demonstrated on blood or X-ray tests.

Patient: *do you think I'm mad?*

Doctor: no, I haven't said that. I don't know what's causing your pain, but you are right that psychological problems can sometimes present in this way and are a potential cause for stomach pain. They do need to be considered in order to enable us to get expert help if this is indeed the case.

Patient: *why can't I just have pethidine to make the pain go away?*

Doctor: we do not think that giving you lots of pethidine to mask the problem is going to help us get you better. But if the pain is continuing to be troublesome, then we would be more than happy to obtain specialist advice from the doctors in the pain clinic.

1.4 Acute scenarios

1.4.1 Nausea and vomiting

Scenario

A 77-year-old woman was initially admitted with chest pain, and during the course of investigation is found to have iron-deficiency anaemia. She is given bowel preparation for a colonoscopy and starts to vomit. You are asked to assess her.

Introduction

There are many causes of nausea and vomiting: serious causes must be excluded rapidly, but thorough consideration of the patient's medical and drug history may be needed to make a diagnosis.

Nausea and vomiting are very common non-specific symptoms that occur in many medical situations. Nausea is a feeling of inclination to vomit and may be associated with hypersalivation and/or regurgitation of small amounts of material from the stomach. Vomiting is not always associated with nausea. Both may be stimulated via many mechanisms within the body, ranging from the higher centres (eg unpleasant visual stimulus) to toxic causes (eg chemotherapeutic agents) to mechanical causes (eg intestinal obstruction). Table 16 shows causes of nausea and vomiting classified with respect to mechanism.

The scenario described is very suggestive of intestinal obstruction that has been precipitated by the bowel preparation, but it is important to consider other causes. Some preparations used for bowel preparation have an unpleasant taste and many patients experience nausea whilst taking them. There is also a history of chest pain, about which no details are given, but this may be cardiac and hence it will be important to exclude the rare but important diagnosis of painless myocardial infarction presenting with vomiting.

History of the presenting problem

- When did the symptoms start? A long history of recurrent vomiting may suggest that this is an acute-on-chronic exacerbation of a known condition such as diabetic gastropathy. Identifying a temporal association with a procedure, new drug or other event may be crucial in diagnosing the underlying problem.

- What was in the vomitus? Vomit is usually partially digested food mixed with gastric juice. The presence of small amounts of

TABLE 16 CAUSES OF NAUSEA AND VOMITING

Mechanism	Type of problem	Example
Central nervous system	Anxiety Nociceptive event Metabolic changes Raised intracranial pressure Drugs	Prior to procedure Phlebotomy Hyponatraemia Cerebral tumour Chemotherapeutic agents, digoxin, theophyllline, opiates
Balance centre	Labyrinthitis Ménière's disease Benign positional vertigo	Viral infection
Mechanical	Gastric outlet obstruction Intestinal obstruction Dysmotility Impacted foreign body	Antral gastric cancer Caecal carcinoma Diabetic gastropathy Gallstone ileus
Gut receptors	Ingested toxin Infection	Drug side effect, eg digoxin Viral gastroenteritis

blood is not unusual, particularly if there has been considerable retching, but large volumes of blood should lead to consideration of causes of haematemesis (see Section 1.4.3). Bilious vomiting may occur in patients who have had previous gastric bypass surgery. Vomiting of food from several meals ago may suggest gastric stasis or gastric outlet obstruction.

- What was the volume of the vomitus? Large-volume vomiting occurs in small bowel obstruction.

- Is there any abdominal pain? Abdominal pain and vomiting should lead to consideration of other specific causes such as peptic ulceration, acute pancreatitis or perforated viscus (see Section 1.4.4). Radiation of the pain towards the chest or down the arms would raise suspicions of a cardiac cause.

- Has there been any change in bowel habit? This may suggest serious underlying pathology such as colonic neoplasia but is also seen in patients with infective gastroenteritis.

- Has the patient passed stool/flatus? Reduced bowel opening or absolute constipation is suggestive of intestinal obstruction.

Intestinal obstruction leads to different symptoms depending on the level of the block.

- Oesophageal obstruction: dysphagia and inability to swallow saliva.
- Gastric obstruction: may cause vomiting with little or no pain.
- Small intestinal obstruction: usually causes vomiting, but the colon may still function.
- Colonic obstruction: often causes pain and constipation, but vomiting may be a late feature.

- Is there any associated dizziness, light-headedness, tinnitus or change in conscious level? These may indicate a central cause for nausea/vomiting from either the vestibular system or central nervous system, but may also suggest severe fluid depletion leading to impaired cerebral perfusion.

Other relevant history

Has there been any previous abdominal surgery, which could lead to adhesions that might cause intestinal obstruction? Does the patient have any other medical or surgical conditions? She was admitted with chest pain, which might be attributable to angina provoked by anaemia, and since acute intestinal obstruction may require surgical intervention it is very important to identify comorbid risks such as ischaemic heart disease at an early stage.

It will be important to ask carefully about current medications and any recent changes in these: drugs are a common cause of nausea and vomiting, and patients taking drugs that affect vascular responses (eg beta-blockers) may be susceptible to smaller losses in circulating volume than would otherwise be the case.

An alcohol history is also important: alcohol excess/abuse is associated with nausea and vomiting, as are many of its complications (eg acute pancreatitis).

Examination

General features

Does the patient look well, ill, very ill or nearly dead? If the latter, then urgent attention and intervention are required. Get senior help early: an experienced hand carries extra authority when negotiating with other colleagues, eg in intensive care or surgical services, and is also important when decisions to limit intervention are appropriate.

If the patient is *in extremis*, summon the cardiac arrest team: do not wait for the heart to stop. Often more can usefully be done in the 'peri-arrest' period than after a cardiac arrest.

- Check vital signs: look in particular for evidence of volume depletion (cool peripheries, tachycardia, hypotension/postural hypotension, low JVP) and of sepsis, which can cause vomiting. Check pulse oximetry.

> If the patient is peripherally shut down and hypotensive, insert two large-bore cannulae and start resuscitation immediately whilst completing the history and examination.

- Check Glasgow Coma Scale (GCS) score: reduction in conscious level may occur in the very ill or it may indicate the underlying cause of vomiting (eg intracerebral lesion). Patients in coma (GCS <8/15) need definitive airway protection as they are at high risk of aspiration of gastric contents.

Given the clinical suspicion of possible malignancy, look for clubbing, cachexia and lymphadenopathy. General examination should also focus on any significant comorbidities that might influence or preclude subsequent investigations or treatments.

> Never lose sight of the whole patient: after initial resuscitation do not focus exclusively on the main problem.

Abdomen
Systematically consider the following.

- Inspection: scars (consider adhesions), distension, abnormal bruising (Cullen's or Grey Turner's sign in acute severe pancreatitis).

- Palpation: signs of peritonism, abdominal mass.

- Auscultation: high-pitched bowel sounds (obstruction); absent bowel sounds (perforation); succussion splash (gastric outlet obstruction).

- Digital rectal examination: presence of malaena, mass lesion or faecal impaction.

Investigation
The appropriate strategy for investigation will clearly depend on the clinical context: the patient who begins to vomit after being given a new medication may not require any investigation at all, but in the scenario described the following would be appropriate.

Routine blood tests

- Check FBC.

- Electrolytes, renal/liver/bone profiles, amylase: may sometimes reveal the cause of nausea and vomiting (eg hyponatraemia, hypercalcaemia) or its effects (eg hypokalaemia); useful in estimating the degree of dehydration, when urea is proportionally elevated to a greater extent than creatinine, also in excluding acute (or acute-on-chronic) renal impairment; abnormal liver blood tests may suggest a biliary cause for vomiting; elevated amylase would clearly raise suspicion of acute pancreatitis.

Routine imaging tests
An erect CXR should be performed in those with abdominal pain to exclude a perforation by looking for free air under the diaphragm, and may also reveal evidence of aspiration pneumonia. A plain abdominal radiograph is essential in those whose vomiting might be due to intestinal obstruction, as in this case (Fig. 10).

Other tests
Given the patient's history of chest pain, a 12-lead ECG should be performed to look for evidence of myocardial ischaemia, and this may need repeating after 8–12 hours to assess for evolving changes; also check serum troponin.

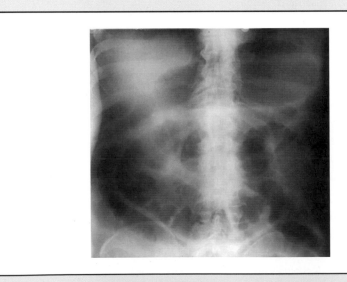

▲ **Fig. 10** Plain abdominal radiograph showing dilated stomach and small bowel in a patient with colonic obstruction.

Other investigations will be determined by the clinical context and the results of preliminary tests. Arterial blood gas analysis is required in any patient who is very ill and may reveal metabolic alkalosis if vomiting has been long-standing. Other structural investigations may be useful in selected cases.

- Ultrasound scanning: particularly good for imaging the gallbladder and proximal biliary tree and can be useful in excluding intra-abdominal fluid collections.

- CT scanning: increasingly used in the investigation of acute abdominal pathology; particularly useful in imaging the pancreas and distal biliary tree but can also reveal other gastrointestinal or non-gastrointestinal pathology.

- Endoscopic retrograde cholangiopancreatography (ERCP)/magnetic resonance cholangiopancreatography (MRCP): imaging of the biliary tree by these techniques may be required in some specific settings, eg acute gallstone pancreatitis, where emergency ERCP with duct drainage is essential in reducing further complications. This should preferably be performed within the first 24 hours as oedema at the papilla worsens over time, reducing the likelihood of successful intervention and increasing the risk of ERCP-related complications.

- Contrast studies: patients with persisting symptoms may require either barium meal or small bowel enema/enteroclysis, which can give information relating to the extent of strictures in the small intestine in addition to assessment of the degree of small bowel obstruction.

> If in doubt, get a surgical opinion: this can wait until blood test results and preliminary imaging studies are available if the patient is not very ill, but if the patient is shocked call for advice as soon as resuscitation is underway.

> Upper gastrointestinal endoscopy contributes little to the investigation of nausea and vomiting (without haematemesis) and is not without risk: the patient may have a stomach full of fluid, increasing the risk of aspiration and reducing the chance of visualising any significant pathology.

Management

Specific management will clearly be dictated by the particular cause of vomiting, but there are three main areas to consider in the management of all patients with this symptom: resuscitation, control of pain, and control of nausea and vomiting.

Resuscitation

> Resuscitation is the most important aspect of immediate management. If the patient is shocked, ie has cool peripheries, tachycardia, hypotension or severe postural hypotension (lying and sitting) and a low JVP, then give high-flow oxygen and:
>
> - insert large-bore cannulae into both forearms/antecubital fossae;
> - give a rapid fluid bolus (1 L of 0.9% saline or colloid);
> - check peripheral perfusion, pulse rate, BP and JVP in response to fluid bolus;
> - if there is still evidence of hypovolaemia, give another rapid fluid bolus;

> - repeat until the peripheries are warming, pulse is settling, BP is restored (without postural drop) and JVP can be seen;
> - insert urinary catheter to monitor urine output.

> Many doctors worry about administering fluid boluses, particularly in the elderly or in those with a history of heart failure. It is true that both groups will not cope well with fluid overload, but both tolerate hypovolaemia poorly and so prompt volume replacement is important. Give rapid boluses of 500 mL rather than 1 L and check regularly for signs of fluid overload.

Central venous lines Central venous catheters take time to insert, do not themselves make anyone better, and attempts to insert them are much more likely to cause harm than benefit in a patient who is clearly hypovolaemic.

> Do not attempt to insert an internal jugular or subclavian central line into someone who is obviously hypovolaemic. When they have been resuscitated a central line may aid continuing fluid management.

Pain control

Patients with pain should be given sufficient analgesia. If they are vomiting, then the drug should be delivered by a parenteral route, either intramuscularly/intravenously or subcutaneously depending on the circumstances. Opiates titrated to the level of adequate analgesia will often be necessary for severe pain.

MMC Core Curriculum   35

⚠ Opiates cause nausea and vomiting in many patients and should therefore always be administered with an antiemetic.

Control of nausea and vomiting

Control of nausea and vomiting is best achieved by identifying the underlying cause and treating this specifically. However, in most cases the exact cause may not be instantly obvious or there may be delay in obtaining relevant information, in which case effective symptom control depends on determining the mechanism or mechanisms of nausea and vomiting in the particular case and selecting the relevant therapeutic intervention

(Fig. 11 and Table 17). In the patient who is nauseous but not vomiting oral medication may be sufficient, but once the patient starts to vomit this route is no longer viable.

🔑 Insertion of a nasogastric tube may be necessary to relieve the symptoms of large-volume vomiting and also allows accurate measurement of fluid loss.

Other useful drug therapies include hyoscine butylbromide, which can be employed to reduce intestinal secretions, and octreotide may be used in a similar fashion. These drugs are used most commonly in patients with complications of advanced cancer.

1.4.2 Acute diarrhoea

Scenario

A 22-year-old man who has just returned from a trip to Thailand is sent to the Emergency Department by ambulance after being seen by the out-of-hours GP service. He looks acutely unwell and is barely responsive to your questions, saying that he has had 'terrible diarrhoea' for several days.

Introduction

This is an emergency: the patient seems to be suffering circulatory failure and neurological disturbance. In a recently returned traveller from

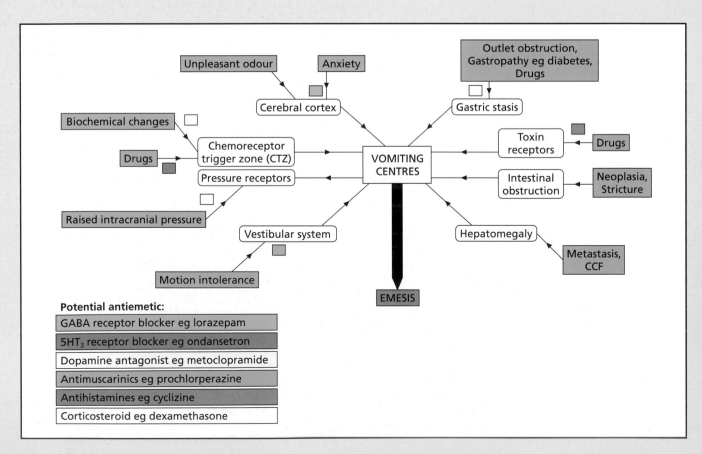

▲**Fig. 11** Pathways involved in nausea and vomiting with specific examples of potential antiemetics for relevant pathways.

TABLE 17 ANTIEMETIC DRUGS AND RECOMMENDED DOSAGE

Antiemetic drug	Dosage per 24 hours
Anxiolytics Lorazepam	4 mg
Dopamine antagonists Metoclopramide Domperidone Haloperidol Levomepromazine (methotrimeprazine)	30–80 mg 30–80 mg 1.5–10 mg 12.5–75 mg
5HT₃ receptor antagonists Ondansetron	8–16 mg
Antimuscarinics Prochlorperazine	5–30 mg
Antihistamines Cyclizine	50–150 mg
Steroids Dexamethasone	8–20 mg

abroad with severe diarrhoea the most likely diagnosis is an acute infection such as bacterial dysentery, although the other conditions listed in Table 18 require consideration.

History of the presenting problem

The patient cannot give a detailed or reliable history, but from any source available (family, friends, GP letter, ambulance crew notes) try to ascertain the following.

- Travel: when did the patient return from abroad, how long was he there, and what precisely was he doing?

- Diarrhoea: when did it start, how many times today and what is it like? Is the diarrhoea watery, suggesting a non-invasive organism such as *Giardia*, *Cryptosporidium* or cholera, or bloody, suggesting bacterial or amoebic dysentery or inflammatory bowel disease?

- Other symptoms: vomiting, fever.

- Have travelling companions been similarly affected? This would make an infective cause very likely.

- Medications: antidiarrhoeal agents may prevent the natural expulsion of stool and can worsen bacterial dysentery; use of antibiotics may result in antibiotic-associated diarrhoea and psuedomembranous colitis caused by *C. difficile* infection; has the patient taken antimalarial prophylaxis (and if so, what)?

Other relevant history

Is there any possibility that the patient may have a non-infectious cause of diarrhoea: has he ever had any similar problems before, which would suggest that inflammatory bowel disease might be the diagnosis? Does he have any pre-existing medical condition such as diabetes, immunodeficiency (including HIV infection) or relevant family history of illness, eg of inflammatory bowel disease? Was the patient vaccinated against *Salmonella* and cholera before travelling?

> ⚠ Just because a patient has been abroad, do not assume that it must be an infectious condition.

Examination

General features

> 🔑 Get help from the intensive care unit urgently if the patient looks very ill or nearly dead.

- Vital signs: look in particular for evidence of intravascular volume depletion (cool peripheries, tachycardia, hypotension/postural

TABLE 18 CAUSES OF SEVERE DIARRHOEA IN THE RETURNING TRAVELLER

Type of cause	Condition
Enteral infection	Bacterial: *Campylobacter*, *Salmonella*, *Shigella*, *Escherichia coli*, *Vibrio cholerae* (if travel to an endemic area), *Clostridium difficile* Protozoal: amoebic dysentery, cryptosporidiosis, giardiasis Viral: rotavirus, Norwalk agent (CMV in the immunocompromised)
Systemic infection with diarrhoeal component	Malaria, pneumonia (especially atypical), septicaemia, meningitis
Non-infectious	Inflammatory bowel disease, drug side effects (especially antibiotics), laxative overuse

CMV, cytomegalovirus.

hypotension, low JVP) and dehydration (reduced skin turgor, dry mucosae). Check pulse oximetry.

> **If resuscitation is required, start immediately.**

- Systemic signs of sepsis: skin rash, which may accompany typhoid fever and Gram-negative sepsis from bacterial dysentery. Is the body temperature abnormally high or low, both of which can be signs of sepsis? Uveitis or arthritis can complicate dysentery.

- Glasgow Coma Scale (GSC) score: is the fact that the patient barely responds to questions the result of general debilitation or does it indicate pathology such as cerebral malaria or meningitis?

Abdomen

Is the abdomen tender or distended? This might indicate colonic dilatation, and possibly precede perforation. Are the liver and spleen enlarged or tender? Bacterial dysentery may result in splenomegaly, while amoebiasis can be associated with liver abscess.

Is the rectal examination normal or is there a bloody or purulent discharge? This indicates probable dysentery or inflammatory bowel disease, and once the patient is stabilised rigid sigmoidoscopy should be considered to obtain a tissue diagnosis.

Investigation

> **Always check thick films for malaria in a patient returning from the tropics with a febrile illness.**

Routine blood tests

- FBC looking for anaemia, leucocytosis, thrombocytopenia: a possible feature of sepsis but also consider haemolytic–uraemic syndrome caused by *E. coli* 0157.

- Electrolytes (hypokalaemia, hypernatraemia).

- Creatinine/urea (renal function, hydration status).

- Liver function tests.

- Inflammatory markers.

- Blood culture.

Stool

Submit a stool sample for microbiological assessment (microscopy, culture, sensitivity; testing for ova, cysts and parasites; *C. difficile* toxin). A freshly evacuated specimen needs to be examined if amoebiasis is suspected.

Imaging

Abdominal radiograph, looking in particular for colonic dilatation, toxic megacolon being defined as a diameter of the transverse colon >6 cm (Fig. 12).

Sigmoidoscopy

Rigid sigmoidoscopy with rectal biopsy should be performed if the patient has bloody diarrhoea or is passing mucopus, suggesting dysentery or colitis, and particularly in an immunocompromised individual, where there may be viral colitis (eg caused by CMV) or cryptosporidial infection. This allows direct visualisation of colonic mucosa and biopsy (see Fig. 4).

Other investigations

The need for other investigations is determined by clinical progress and the results of routine testing, eg serological tests for amoebiasis and yersiniosis (also for coeliac disease) may be appropriate.

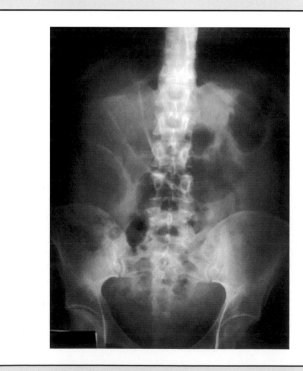

▲ **Fig. 12** Plain abdominal radiograph showing a very dilated colon (toxic megacolon).

Management

🔑 In a sick patient with an acute diarrhoeal/colitic illness, start treatment before the results of tests are available.

- Resuscitate: as described in Section 1.4.1.
- Ciprofloxacin (500 mg iv bd) and metronidazole (500 mg iv tds): to treat presumed bacterial or amoebic dysentery.
- Hydrocortisone (200 mg iv qds): to cover possibility of inflammatory bowel disease.
- Surgical review: in case there is actual or impending colonic perforation.

⚠️ Obtain a surgical opinion (preferably from an experienced gastroenterological surgeon) immediately if there is peritonism or the abdominal radiograph shows toxic megacolon or free air, or if patient does not improve rapidly with rehydration and the treatment listed above. Emergency colectomy may be required.

Further comments

Is there a public health issue: are others affected, and was the airline's caterer rather than the roadside food vendor in Bangkok to blame?

🔑 **Public health issues**

- Food poisoning and dysentery cases should be notified to the Public Health Laboratory Service, which will consider instigating case-finding and source-tracing of any outbreak.
- The attending doctor could reasonably offer testing and treatment to known contacts of the index case.

🔑 If dealing with acute gastroenteritis 'in the field', remember the World Health Organization/UNICEF oral rehydration fluid: 1 L water, 10 g (2 teaspoons) sugar, 2.5 g ($^1/_2$ teaspoon) salt, 2.5 g ($^1/_2$ teaspoon) baking soda (sodium bicarbonate).

1.4.3 Haematemesis and melaena

Scenario

A 75-year-old man is brought by ambulance to the Emergency Department after he collapsed after walking to the bathroom, where he vomited some blood. He gives a history of melaena over the last 2 days.

Introduction

Haematemesis is due to bleeding from the oesophagus, stomach or duodenum; it is very unusual for bleeding distal to the duodenojejunal junction to return to the stomach. The history of melaena (dark tarry faeces containing blood) indicates the patient has had a gastrointestinal haemorrhage from a lesion anywhere from the oesophagus to the terminal ileum (Table 19), with the most likely cause being peptic ulceration. More distal haemorrhage results in fresh rectal bleeding, although occasional patients with caecal malignancies present with melaena.

Important issues are to determine the severity of the haemorrhage, the likely cause of bleeding, and whether there is continued bleeding. It is also important to assess for the presence of comorbidities such as a chronic liver disease or ischaemic heart disease, which increase the mortality associated with gastrointestinal bleeding.

History of the presenting problem

- Nature of the vomit: find out if this was fresh blood, which suggests a proximal source of bleeding (eg oesophagus), a large gastrointestinal haemorrhage or persistent bleeding, or was 'coffee grounds', suggestive of altered and therefore old blood. Patients who say 'it might have looked a bit like coffee grounds' are extremely unlikely to have had significant gastrointestinal bleeding and should be managed as if vomiting is the problem rather than haematemesis (see Section 1.4.1).

- Quantity of blood loss: patients are most unlikely to be able to give a more precise estimate than

TABLE 19 DIFFERENTIAL DIAGNOSIS OF MELAENA		
Common	**Less common**	**Rare**
Duodenal ulceration	Oesophageal/gastric varices	Aortoenteric fistulae[2]
Gastric ulceration/erosions	Dieulafoy lesion[1]	Small bowel tumour
Gastric carcinoma	Angiodysplasia	
NSAID-induced enteropathy		
Oesophagitis		

1. Bleeding from an arteriole protruding through a minute mucosal defect, usually in the proximal stomach.
2. Rare complication of abdominal aortic aneurysm repair, very rare in other circumstances.

that there was a 'lot' or a 'little'. Dizziness or syncope suggests significant bleeding.

🔑 Syncope suggests a significant gastrointestinal haemorrhage or a lesser bleed against the background of chronic anaemia.

⚠️ Persistent life-threatening bleeding can occur with melaena in the absence of haematemesis.

- Vomiting before bleeding: recurrent or forceful vomiting followed by haematemesis typically occurs with a Mallory–Weiss tear. A peptic ulcer in the pyloric canal causing gastric outflow obstruction may cause vomiting after eating before melaena.

- Abdominal pain: recent retrosternal discomfort with acid reflux into the mouth suggests oesophagitis. Gastric and duodenal ulcers may be associated with epigastric discomfort or 'indigestion' and pain radiating through to the back typically occurs with a deep posterior duodenal ulcer. The possibility of perforation must be considered if pain is severe, but it is uncommon for perforation and haematemesis to coexist.

- Weight loss: raises suspicion of an underlying carcinoma but can occur through reduced oral intake due to pain from a peptic ulcer.

Other relevant history

Aside from the obvious point of establishing whether the patient has had any previous episodes of gastrointestinal bleeding and, if so,

what caused them, the key issues to pursue are drug history, the possibility of chronic liver disease, history of previous abdominal surgery, and history of comorbidities.

Drug history

- NSAIDs and aspirin can cause either ulceration or erosions in the stomach, duodenum or small bowel.

- Anticoagulation with warfarin clearly has the potential to make any bleeding worse.

- Beta-blockers may mask a tachycardia associated with hypovolaemia.

Chronic liver disease

Are there any features suggestive of chronic liver disease, which clearly increases the risk of oesophageal or gastric varices? Recognising that some patients may find the necessary questions embarrassing or offensive, explain why you need to know the information: 'Liver disease can cause bleeding like this, so I need to know whether you have liver disease or are at risk of liver disease'. Explore the following.

- History of liver disease: 'Have you ever been told you have cirrhosis, liver disease or a scarred liver? Have you ever been jaundiced? Have you ever had a distended abdomen due to fluid (ascites)?'

- Risk of liver disease: 'The things that put you at risk of liver disease are alcohol and some viruses. Are you at risk of these? How much alcohol do you normally drink? Have you ever been a heavy drinker in the past? Are you at risk of hepatitis B or hepatitis C? The things that put you at risk are blood transfusions, intravenous drug use, and some sexual practices.'

Previous abdominal surgery

If the patient has had surgery for bleeding gastric or duodenal ulcers in the past, then if possible it is important to establish the nature of the operation. Current practice is almost invariably to simply oversew a bleeding ulcer, but formerly a partial gastrectomy with or without a gastroenterostomy (Billroth I or II) used to be performed (Figs 13 and 14). There is an increased incidence of stomal ulceration and carcinoma of the stoma following partial gastrectomy, and knowledge of

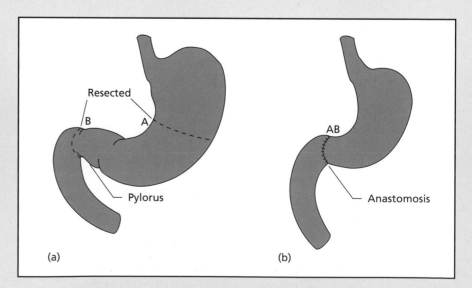

▲ **Fig. 13** Schematic diagram of the anatomy following a partial gastrectomy (Billroth I).

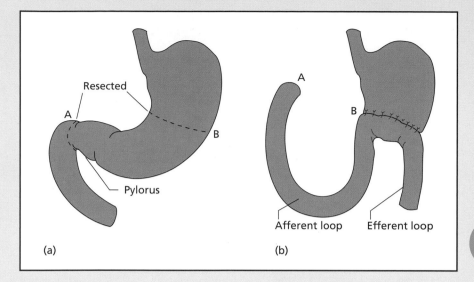

▲**Fig. 14** Schematic diagram of the anatomy following a partial gastrectomy with a gastroenterostomy (Billroth II).

previous intervention aids endoscopic diagnosis.

It is very important to elicit a history of aortic aneurysm surgery: patients with gastrointestinal bleeding and an aortic graft may have an aortoenteric fistula and merit emergency endoscopy and/or cross-sectional imaging.

Comorbidities

The presence of ischaemic heart disease, chronic pulmonary disease and/or organ failure (renal, cardiac or liver) increases the morbidity and mortality associated with gastrointestinal bleeding. Risk scores have been developed to take these into account in determining the management of gastrointestinal bleeding.

Examination

General features

How much blood has the patient lost?

- Cool peripheries: how far up the fingers/hands/arms do you have to feel before the skin feels warm?

- Pulse: tachycardia.
- Hypotension/postural hypotension (lying and sitting): if BP falls significantly on sitting up, then the patient's homeostatic mechanisms are nearly overwhelmed.
- JVP: can you see it?

If resuscitation is required, start immediately.

The severity of the bleeding and risk of death can be assessed clinically on the basis of the patient's age, pulse, systolic BP and comorbidity (Table 20). As would be expected, hypotension (systolic BP <100 mmHg) and tachycardia (pulse >100 bpm) in association with old age and comorbidity indicate a poor prognosis.

⚠ **When dealing with a patient with gastrointestinal bleeding, do not forget to look specifically for features of chronic liver disease (see Section 1.2.2) and for evidence of hepatic encephalopathy (see Section 1.4.6).**

Abdomen

Apart from confirming the presence of melaena on rectal examination, abdominal examination will be normal in most cases of gastrointestinal bleeding, but check for any abdominal mass and for features of portal hypertension/chronic liver disease (see Section 1.2.2).

TABLE 20 CLINICAL ASSESSMENT OF THE SEVERITY OF GASTROINTESTINAL HAEMORRHAGE BASED ON INITIAL CLINICAL FINDINGS PRIOR TO ENDOSCOPY (ROCKALL SCORE)

Clinical parameter	Score			
	0	1	2	3
Age (years)	<60	60–79	>80	
Shock				
Systolic BP (mmHg)	<100	>100	<100	
Pulse (bpm)	<100	>100		
Comorbidity	Nil	Other	Cardiac failure IHD	Renal failure Liver failure
Total score	0	2	4	6
Mortality (%)	0.2	5	24	49

IHD, ischaemic heart disease.

Investigation

 Immediately organise cross-match of at least 4 units of blood for anyone who appears to have had a substantial gastrointestinal bleed.

Routine blood tests

FBC (haemoglobin, mean corpuscular volume: reduced in chronic iron-deficiency anaemia), electrolytes, creatinine/urea (urea is elevated out of proportion to creatinine due to blood in the bowel), liver function tests, clotting screen.

The haemoglobin may initially be normal following an acute gastrointestinal bleed. However, a normal haemoglobin should not be reassuring in the patient who is tachycardic and hypotensive and the value should be rechecked after 8–12 hours.

Gastrointestinal endoscopy

Upper gastrointestinal endoscopy is useful in the management of upper gastrointestinal bleeding but does not replace adequate resuscitation and management of comorbid illnesses.

It is dangerous to perform endoscopy on a patient who is hypovolaemic.

Upper gastrointestinal endoscopy should ideally be performed within 24 hours of admission in anyone with a substantial gastrointestinal bleed. Urgent endoscopy is indicated if oesophageal varices are suspected or the patient continues to bleed actively. It may be necessary for this to be performed in theatre with the surgical team on 'standby', when endoscopy will hopefully define the lesion and also exclude variceal haemorrhage or an inoperable gastric cancer (Figs 15–17).

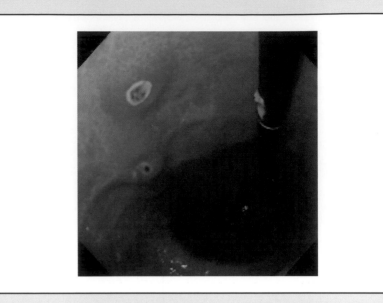

▲ **Fig. 15** Small gastric ulcer and adjacent erosion viewed at gastroscopy.

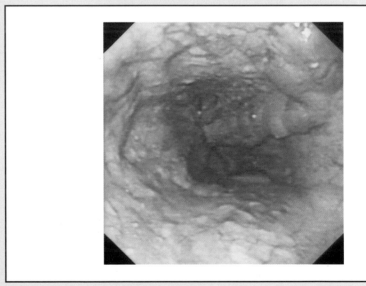

▲ **Fig. 16** Small oesophageal varices.

Endoscopic stigmata of recent haemorrhage

- Blood in the stomach.
- Clot over an ulcer.
- Actively bleeding vessel.

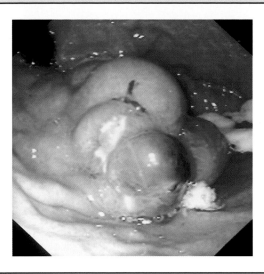

▲ **Fig. 17** Varices at the gastro-oesophageal junction with surface ulceration and clot.

Endoscopic stigmata of recent haemorrhage help in stratifying risk of rebleeding and mortality. If an adherent clot is seen in a peptic ulcer, there is a 20% chance of rebleed; if a visible vessel is seen in a peptic ulcer, there is up to a 50% chance of rebleeding; if neither of these are found, then the chance of rebleeding is <10%. Endoscopy will be normal in 30% of patients with suspected upper gastrointestinal bleeds. Ongoing bleeding should always prompt consideration of repeat endoscopy as small bleeding points can be missed.

Radiological imaging

Most patients with gastrointestinal bleeding do not require radiological tests. An abdominal radiograph is almost never indicated. An erect CXR is appropriate if a perforation is suspected (free air under the diaphragm), if the patient has vomited and there is the possibility of aspiration pneumonia, or if required for anaesthetic assessment prior to theatre. In the very rare circumstance of the patient with an abdominal aortic graft and the possibility of an aortoenteric fistula, then CT of the abdomen may be indicated.

Management

> 🔑 **Management of the patient with gastrointestinal haemorrhage**
>
> - Resuscitate first, ask questions afterwards.
> - Early liaison with the surgical team.

> ⚠️ If the patient is shocked, ie has cool peripheries, tachycardia, hypotension or severe postural hypotension (lying and sitting) and a low JVP, then give high-flow oxygen and:
>
> - insert large-bore cannulae into both forearms/antecubital fossae;
> - give a rapid fluid bolus of 1 L of 0.9% saline or colloid, or 2 units blood (O negative or cross-matched) if available;
> - check peripheral perfusion, pulse rate, BP and JVP in response to fluid bolus;
> - if there is still evidence of hypovolaemia, give more blood;
> - repeat until the peripheries are warming, pulse is settling, BP is restored (without postural drop) and JVP can be seen;
> - insert urinary catheter to monitor urine output.

Venous access

> 🔑 If you cannot establish peripheral venous access in a patient with gastrointestinal bleeding, then cannulate the femoral vein, which lies medial to the femoral artery (remembered by the acronym 'NAVY': nerve, artery, vein and Y-fronts). Do not attempt to insert an internal jugular or subclavian line.

Resuscitation is the most important aspect of management: remember that a central line, like an endoscopy, does not replace adequate resuscitation, so do not attempt to insert one into a patient who is clearly hypovolaemic. A central line never made anyone better in this circumstance but has killed quite a few: insertion is difficult when veins are constricted, making the chance of complications much higher, and knowing exactly how low the CVP is will not alter management.

Once intravascular volume has been restored, a central line should be considered in the following situations:

- hypotensive on admission and age over 60 years;

- rebled;

- if transfusion requirements exceed 4 units;

- accompanying severe cardiorespiratory or renal disease;

- initial Rockall score ≥2 (in patient under 60 years of age) or ≥3 (in patients over 60 years of age).

> ⚠️ Diagnosing rebleeding is not always straightforward but is suggested by:
>
> - overt fresh haematemesis or melaena, although melaena can persist for a few days following a bleed;

- development of new tachycardia of >100 bpm with drop of systolic BP to <90 mmHg;
- development of new tachycardia of >100 bpm with fall in CVP;
- drop in haemoglobin concentration of >2 g/dL over a period of 24 hours or less.

TABLE 21 THE MOST COMMON CAUSES OF HAEMATEMESIS IN PATIENTS WITH LIVER CIRRHOSIS

Cause	Frequency (%)
Bleeding oesophageal varices	60
Bleeding peptic ulcer	20
Portal hypertensive gastropathy	5
Bleeding gastric varices	5
Other causes and undiagnosed	10

Is surgical or radiological intervention required?

Inform surgical colleagues sooner rather than later: as a 'rule of thumb' discuss any patient who merits emergency endoscopy, has an initial Rockall score over 3 or requires significant transfusion. The decision regarding the appropriateness and timing of surgery can be very difficult and should be made by experienced, senior colleagues. Early surgery, especially in older patients, is associated with a lower overall mortality and may be indicated for those who meet criteria such as:

- transfusion requirements of >8 units (age <60 years) or >4 units (age >60 years) in 24 hours; or

- one rebleed; or

- spurting vessel at endoscopy not controlled by injection therapy; or

- continued bleeding.

Interventional radiology may be appropriate and should also be explored in tandem with a surgical consult. It has a particularly important role in those with significant comorbidities associated with poor postoperative outcomes.

Other treatments

There is no strong evidence for the initiation of acid suppression until after an endoscopic diagnosis has been made. High-dose intravenous proton pump inhibitor reduces rebleeding in those who have received endoscopic treatment of

bleeding peptic ulcers (eg omeprazole 80 mg iv bolus followed by infusion at 8 mg/hour). Similarly, oral proton pump inhibitors may be indicated for oesophagitis or in the healing of a documented ulcer. Eradication of *Helicobacter pylori* is indicated if infection is present with a gastric or duodenal ulcer.

Any clotting disorder should be corrected, and if significant gastrointestinal haemorrhage occurs in a patient on aspirin or warfarin, the risk–benefit for continued use of these medications should be considered carefully.

Further comments

Bleeding from oesophageal varices

> Upper gastrointestinal endoscopy can be both diagnostic and therapeutic in the patient with bleeding oesophageal varices and should be performed as soon as it is safe to do so when these are suspected.

A large-volume painless haematemesis is very suspicious of oesophageal variceal bleeding, particularly if there is any indication of chronic liver disease. However, portal hypertension and variceal haemorrhage may occur in patients without cirrhosis, eg as a result of portal vein thrombosis (see

Section 1.2.2), and also remember that other causes of bleeding, particularly peptic ulcer disease, can and do occur in the context of portal hypertension (Table 21).

Variceal haemorrhage is a life-threatening emergency: patients are at risk of further bleeding, particularly immediately following an initial haemorrhage, and the overall mortality in the short and long term is high. As for any other cause of gastrointestinal bleeding the immediate priority is to recognise shock and resuscitate. Other aspects of management are detailed below.

Treatments to stop bleeding
The following therapies should be considered for those with variceal bleeding.

- Pharmacological measures to reduce variceal haemorrhage by reducing splanchnic blood flow: octreotide and vasopressin analogues (eg terlipressin 2 mg iv 4-hourly) should be used when variceal haemorrhage is suspected.

- Correction of haemostatic/clotting abnormalities: patients with decompensated cirrhosis typically have low platelet counts and a prolonged prothrombin time. It is usual practice to attempt to correct any concomitant vitamin K deficiency, to maintain platelet counts above 50×10^9/L, and to transfuse 2 units of fresh frozen

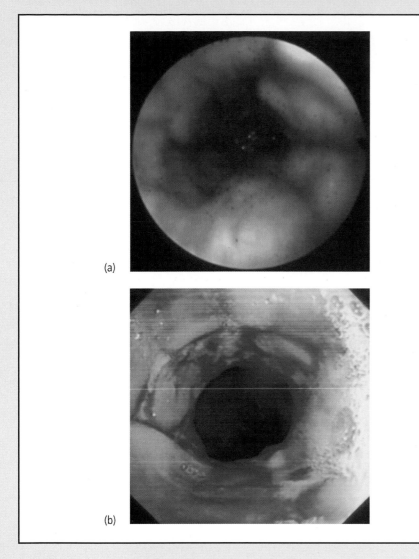

(a)

(b)

▲ **Fig. 18** Oesophageal varices: **(a)** large varices; **(b)** banded varices with superficial banding ulcers.

performed with radiological guidance and is particularly valuable for cases where bleeding is from gastric or ectopic varices, which can be difficult or impossible to control by other means.

- Emergency surgery: rarely indicated, but surgical shunts (eg splenorenal) are occasionally performed (eg for bleeding in the presence of portal vein thrombosis or failed TIPSS insertion). Surgical transection of the oesophagus is now very seldom, if ever, practised.

⚠ **Rebleeding from varices**

Patients remain at increased risk of rebleeding for about 7 days, when their risk returns to that of any patient with chronic liver disease and portal hypertension. It is therefore usual to monitor patients in hospital, and to maintain infusions of octreotide or a vasopressin analogue for 48 hours after acute haemorrhage has been controlled.

In the longer term, patients with oesophageal varices should be enrolled in a programme of endoscopic variceal obliteration using sclerotherapy or band ligation. Where these measures fail, elective surgical or radiological (TIPSS) shunting should be considered, and also liver transplantation in selected cases.

Other treatments The following additional therapies should also be considered.

🔑 Variceal haemorrhage may precipitate more widespread hepatic decompensation with ascites, jaundice, coagulopathy and encephalopathy (see Section 1.4.6).

plasma for every 4 units of blood or packed cells.

- Endoscopic therapy: both diagnostic and therapeutic; should be performed as soon as it is safe to do so. Bleeding oesophageal varices may be injected with sclerosant or ligated with rubber bands to stem bleeding (Fig. 18).

- Balloon tamponade: when haemorrhage is torrential or other factors prevent effective and safe emergency endoscopy, balloon tamponade of the gastric fundus and oesophagus may achieve haemostasis. A Sengstaken–

Blakemore or Minnesota tube is employed in some specialist units as a temporary measure (Fig. 19). This should not be used continuously for longer than 24 hours, risks including inadvertent intubation of the trachea and oesophageal perforation.

- Emergency transjugular intrahepatic portosystemic shunt (TIPSS): reserved for those failing endoscopic treatment. Reduces portal hypertension by deploying a stent to maintain a shunt between the portal vein and a major hepatic vein. The procedure is

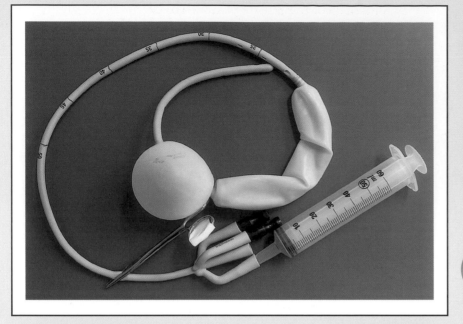

▲**Fig. 19** Sengstaken–Blakemore tube. This particular tube has a gastric (inflated) balloon, an oesophageal (deflated) balloon, a gastric aspiration channel and an oesophageal aspiration channel. In most cases tamponade can be achieved by just inflating the gastric balloon. The gastro-oesophageal junction is 40 cm from the mouth.

1.4.4 Acute abdominal pain

> ### Scenario
>
> A 44-year-old woman is admitted to the Emergency Department with a 12-hour history of severe abdominal pain. Her husband called the ambulance because she seemed to be getting confused.

Introduction

> 🔑 Physicians need to know how to manage a patient with abdominal pain, even if this is traditionally regarded as a surgical problem.

Consider the possible causes of abdominal pain given in Table 22.

> 🔑 Is the patient ill, very ill or nearly dead? What are the vital signs? Are there signs of peritonitis? Your initial assessment should be complete in a few minutes. Start resuscitation immediately. Call for surgical assistance without delay if there is shock or peritonitis. Do not delay treatment chasing irrelevant minutiae.

- Antibiotics: there is an association of bleeding oesophageal varices with sepsis, and patients are at risk of aspiration pneumonia, so it is standard practice to administer broad-spectrum antibiotics after performing a septic screen (eg cefotaxime 1 g iv twice daily). Ascites frequently develops over a period of 3–5 days in patients who have had a variceal haemorrhage, and prophylactic antibiotics on admission also reduce the risk of spontaneous bacterial peritonitis.

- Laxatives (lactulose) and enemas: are essential to reduce the risk of hepatic encephalopathy, which is aggravated by the enteric protein load of blood.

- Nutrition: patients with chronic liver disease are often malnourished and should be allowed to eat as soon as possible. Protein restriction is rarely indicated. Sodium intake should be less than 100 mmol/day, which can be achieved most simply by not adding salt to food at the table. Thiamine replacement should be used where there is a history of excess alcohol use.

- Avoidance of alcohol withdrawal: a reducing regimen of a benzodiazepine should be prescribed if appropriate, eg chlordiazepoxide 30 mg qds on day 1, gradually reducing to none on day 7.

TABLE 22 DIFFERENTIAL DIAGNOSIS OF SEVERE ABDOMINAL PAIN[1]

Common	Less common	Rare
Acute appendicitis	Perforated peptic ulcer	Gastric volvulus
Biliary colic/acute cholecystitis	Acute diverticulitis	Myocardial infarction[2]
Small bowel obstruction	Intestinal infarction	Lower lobe pneumonia[2]
Acute pancreatitis	Renal colic	Other medical causes, eg
Acute gynaecological disease (including ectopic pregnancy)	Leaking abdominal aortic aneurysm	diabetes, herpes zoster (before the rash), acute porphyria (very rare)

1. In up to one-third of cases no clear diagnosis will be made.
2. Rarely present with abdominal pain.

History of the presenting problem

The patient is not likely to be able to give a detailed history, and trying to extract one is unlikely to be rewarding. Focus on the key issues.

Type of pain

Pancreatic pain is usually constant, epigastric and radiates through to the back. Peptic ulcer pain is often similar, and there may well be a preceding history of indigestion, but pain in the back would be an unusual feature unless the ulcer involves the posterior wall of the duodenum. Biliary pain is typically colicky, often focused in the right upper quadrant and epigastrium, and there may be radiation to the shoulder or shoulder blade due to diaphragmatic irritation. Small bowel disease (obstruction or infarction) is usually associated with central or low abdominal pain, whilst renal colic typically affects the loin area (sometimes with classic radiation to the groin). Appendicitis typically begins with central colicky abdominal pain that then moves to the right iliac fossa. Rarely thoracic problems can present as an acute abdomen, so remember to check for radiation in a cardiac pattern, and for symptoms suggestive of pneumonia.

Onset and duration of the problem

Sudden onset of epigastric pain would suggest perforation of a peptic ulcer. Most acute abdomens present within 24 hours of onset of symptoms. Biliary colic may occasionally present with a more prolonged prodrome, including discoloration of urine (indicating biliary obstruction) and fevers/rigors (indicating acute cholecystitis/cholangitis). There may be a preceding history of increasing dyspepsia with peptic ulcer disease. A myocardial infarction may present on a background of increasing angina. An infarcted bowel may be preceded by symptoms of mesenteric angina (postprandial epigastric pain and weight loss).

Vomiting

Haematemesis is most likely to be seen in ulcer disease. Faeculent vomit can be seen in any small bowel obstruction or in severe cases of ileus (including pancreatitis). Be wary of the term 'coffee grounds' and do not talk the patient and the medical team into thinking that the problem is haematemesis: if asked enough times, almost all patients/relatives will eventually say that the vomitus 'did look a bit like coffee grounds'.

Bowels

Absolute constipation (faeces and flatus) suggests bowel obstruction.

Other relevant history

Find out if there is there a history of alcohol excess (associated with acute pancreatitis), gallstone disease (associated with biliary colic, cholangitis and pancreatitis), indigestion/peptic ulcer disease, previous abdominal surgery (may cause adhesions and bowel obstruction), urinary symptoms, gynaecological history/symptoms (when was the last menstrual period, could the woman be pregnant, has there been a vaginal discharge?).

Is the patient taking any antacid preparations or on any ulcerogenic medications, eg aspirin, NSAIDs?

Is there a history of ischaemic heart disease or of symptoms suggestive of unstable angina? Firstly, this might be relevant for diagnosis (atypical presentation with abdominal pain); secondly, the presence of severe coronary disease (or any other major medical comorbidity) could certainly influence management of the patient with abdominal pain of any cause.

Examination

General features

If the patient is nearly dead (unrecordable BP, thready pulse, depressed conscious level), call immediately for help from the intensive care unit.

Young patients can sustain a significant insult before showing obvious signs of cardiovascular compromise, but once they decompensate they can do so very rapidly. Be particularly alert for postural hypotension, which is often a warning that the patient is about to 'go off in a big way'.

- Check vital signs: look in particular for evidence of volume depletion (cool peripheries, tachycardia, hypotension/postural hypotension, low JVP). Check pulse oximetry. Fever might suggest a perforated viscus/peritonitis, acute cholecystitis/cholangitis or pancreatitis, but remember that a very ill patient can be profoundly septic with a normal temperature, or even hypothermia.

If the patient is peripherally shut down and hypotensive, insert two large-bore cannulae and start resuscitation immediately whilst completing the history and examination.

- Check Glasgow Coma Scale (GCS) score: reduction in conscious level indicates significant decrease in cerebral perfusion in this context.

- Other features to look for specifically include jaundice (suggests cholangitis or biliary obstruction), evidence of chronic alcohol use or liver disease (see Section 1.2.2: would increase the likelihood of acute pancreatitis) and evidence of peripheral vascular disease (absent pulses, bruits: would increase the likelihood of intestinal infarction).

> 🔑 The presence of jaundice early on is useful in identifying a biliary cause for an acute abdomen; at a later stage it is much less discriminating.

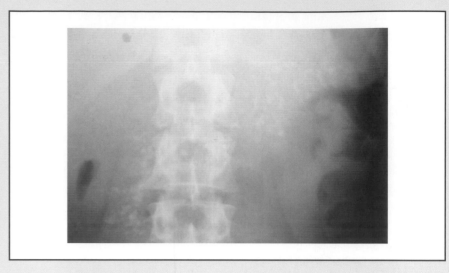

▲**Fig. 20** Plain abdominal radiograph showing pancreatic calcification in a patient with chronic pancreatitis.

Abdomen

> 🔑 Does the patient have peritonitis? If so, call a surgeon immediately.

The presence of generalised tenderness on palpation is to be expected in any patient with acute abdominal pain and is not of great diagnostic help. Far more significant is the presence of guarding and rebound tenderness of localised peritonitis. Is there an abdominal aortic aneurysm? You may not make the diagnosis unless you specifically consider it when palpating the abdomen.

Abdominal distension in this setting is likely to indicate intestinal obstruction or ileus. Pancreatitis can rarely cause ascites, but this would be exceedingly uncommon at presentation. High-pitched tinkling bowel sounds suggest intestinal obstruction; absent bowel sounds suggest ileus. Look for abdominal wall bruising: periumbilical bruising (Cullen's sign) or flank bruising

(Grey Turner's sign) is seen in severe acute pancreatitis.

Rectal examination may reveal tenderness (on the right side with retrocaecal appendicitis) and (rarely in this context) melaena.

Investigation

Routine blood tests
Check FBC (anaemia, leucocytosis), electrolytes, renal/liver/bone profiles, amylase, clotting screen, group and save. An amylase three times the upper limit of the laboratory normal range is diagnostic of acute pancreatitis; lesser elevations are common in other causes of acute abdominal pain and are not diagnostically useful. Check arterial blood gases if the patient is very ill.

Imaging tests
A plain CXR may demonstrate free air under the diaphragm if there is perforation, a pleural effusion (consider pancreatitis as well as chest pathology) or occasionally pneumonia. An abdominal radiograph may show widespread small bowel distension, an isolated (sentinel) loop (associated with acute pancreatitis) or pancreatic

calcification (usually associated with alcoholic chronic pancreatitis, Fig. 20).

Abdominal ultrasound
This may be used to visualise the biliary tree (gallstones, tender thick-walled gallbladder due to cholecystitis, or biliary dilatation) and pancreas (although of limited use in diagnosing pancreatitis). Free intra-abdominal fluid can also be identified.

Abdominal CT scan
The use of CT in acute abdominal pain is becoming more frequent, particularly in the diagnosis of appendicitis (ultrasound is an alternative), small bowel obstruction, acute pancreatitis, as well as in cases of suspected abdominal aortic aneurysm (Fig. 21).

> ⚠ The correct management for the patient with peritonitis is usually an urgent laparotomy: harm can come from delay caused by organisation of unnecessary imaging tests.

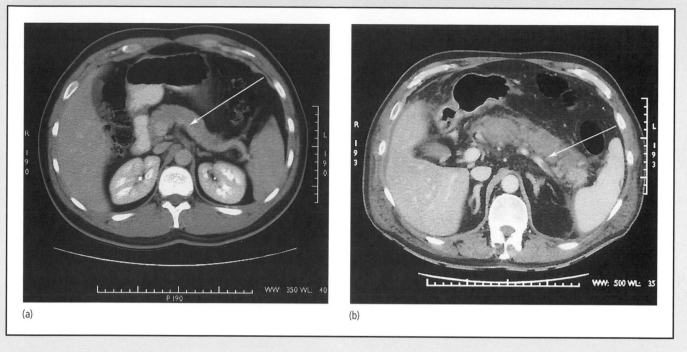

▲**Fig. 21** Abdominal CT scan. (**a**) Normal pancreas (arrow). (**b**) Acute pancreatitis: the pancreas is swollen and oedematous (arrow) and a thrombus can be seen in the splenic vein behind the pancreas (just below point of arrowhead).

Management

> Resuscitation is the most important aspect of immediate management. If the patient is shocked, ie has cool peripheries, tachycardia, hypotension or severe postural hypotension (lying and sitting) and a low JVP, then give high-flow oxygen and:
>
> - insert large-bore cannulae into both forearms/antecubital fossae;
> - give a rapid fluid bolus (1 L of 0.9% saline or colloid);
> - check peripheral perfusion, pulse rate, BP and JVP In response to fluid bolus;
> - if there is still evidence of hypovolaemia, give another rapid fluid bolus;
> - repeat until the peripheries are warming, pulse is settling, BP is restored (without postural drop) and JVP can be seen;
> - insert urinary catheter to monitor urine output.

> The patient with an acute abdomen requires a surgical opinion as soon as resuscitation is underway: surgery may be the definitive treatment.

Pain should be promptly and efficiently relieved with an NSAID, eg diclofenac 75 mg im, or opioid, eg morphine 5 mg sc plus 5 mg im (with antiemetic such as cyclizine 50 mg iv).

Further comments

Management of acute pancreatitis

In some hospitals patients with acute pancreatitis are managed on medical wards by physicians, and many hospitals have their own protocols for doing so. Issues to consider are as follows.

- Analgesia: pethidine is preferred in pancreatitis as morphine may cause spasm of the sphincter of Oddi and worsen the condition.

- Antibiotics: their role in management of acute pancreatitis is unclear. They should always be given if infection is proven, and many would use a second- or third-generation cephalosporin and metronidazole in severely ill patients.

- Nutrition: early feeding is associated with a significant survival benefit in acute pancreatitis. Enteral feeding (oral, nasogastric or nasojejunal) is recommended, but intravenous feeding should be considered early if the gut is not working adequately.

- Endoscopic retrograde cholangiopancreatography: should be considered urgently where there is evidence of cholangitis or if gallstones are implicated in the development of pancreatitis, but after 24 hours of pancreatitis oedema around the ampulla makes this technically very difficult.

Acute pancreatitis may be due to alcohol abuse: be vigilant for signs of alcohol withdrawal and treat this appropriately (see Section 1.4.3).

The presence of persistent pain, fever and raised inflammatory markers may suggest the development of a pancreatic abscess or infection of necrotic pancreatic tissue. These complications, which may require surgical or radiological drainage, are best diagnosed by CT scanning.

After recovery from an attack of gallstone-related pancreatitis, cholecystectomy should be performed when all intra-abdominal inflammation has settled. After recovery from an attack of pancreatitis of any cause abstinence from alcohol is recommended, particularly where alcohol was the precipitating factor, and patient and doctor should be aware of the possibility that both endocrine and exocrine pancreatic insufficiency might develop.

1.4.5 Jaundice

Scenario

A 52-year-old woman with a history of a previous cholecystectomy presents with jaundice of 1 week's duration. This is accompanied by a dull ache in her right upper quadrant. She admits to drinking at least one bottle of wine every other day for the last 2 years.

Introduction

Jaundice in adults is very rarely due to a prehepatic cause (eg haemolysis); hepatic (eg parenchymal disease) or

---

TABLE 23 DIFFERENTIAL DIAGNOSIS OF JAUNDICE DUE TO INTRINSIC LIVER DISEASE

Common	Less common	Rare
Acute alcoholic hepatitis	Acute hepatitis B	Hepatic venous outflow obstruction (Budd–Chiari syndrome, right heart failure)
Acute hepatitis A	Acute hepatitis E	
Drug-induced hepatotoxicity	Autoimmune chronic active hepatitis	Weil's disease
Intrahepatic cholestasis due to sepsis		Wilson's disease
Chronic liver disease		Pregnancy-associated liver disease

TABLE 24 DIFFERENTIAL DIAGNOSIS OF OBSTRUCTIVE JAUNDICE

Common	Less common	Rare
Choledocholithiasis	Cholangiocarcinoma	Primary sclerosing cholangitis
Carcinoma of pancreas	External compression from malignant hilar lymph nodes	
Chronic pancreatitis		

---

posthepatic (eg biliary obstruction) causes are most likely (Tables 23 and 24). History, examination and liver function tests usually give a good indication of which of these broad categories applies to the patient, but liver ultrasound is virtually mandatory. Dilated common and intrahepatic bile ducts indicate obstruction; parenchymal liver disease is more likely if the ducts are normal sized (in the absence of pain).

History of the presenting problem

Not all jaundice in the alcohol abuser is due to alcoholic hepatitis.

Important features to pursue include the following.

- Pain: the presence of pain can indicate obstruction of the common bile duct (CBD) with a stone. Carcinoma of the pancreas

classically presents with painless jaundice. Parenchymal liver disease occasionally results in right upper quadrant discomfort due to stretching of the liver capsule.

Pain is unusual in obstructive jaundice that is not due to CBD stones, but biliary pain must be differentiated from abdominal discomfort that can occur in a case of hepatitis.

- Weight loss: an ominous symptom that may indicate pancreatic carcinoma or cholangiocarcinoma.

- Change in colour of stool and urine: in obstructive jaundice the stool becomes paler (because bile is unable to flow into the intestine and colour the stool) and the urine darker (excess conjugated bilirubin). Remember, however, that similar (though less extreme) changes can also occur in parenchymal disease because inflammation of the liver parenchyma can cause local obstruction of the bile cannaliculi and interlobular bile ducts.

- Fever: together with pain and jaundice forms Charcot's triad, which is characteristic of ascending cholangitis due to bacterial infection in the biliary system. This is usually a complication of CBD stones and rarely occurs with pancreatic carcinoma.

Other relevant history

Alcohol history

The details given in this clinical scenario clearly indicate that alcohol may be the cause of the problem, but this possibility is often concealed. Sometimes a history that includes head injuries, rib or other peripheral fractures, unexplained epileptic seizures, recurrent acute pancreatitis and/or gastrointestinal bleeding can suggest long-standing alcohol excess. Without causing

offence (see *Clinical Skills for PACES*) you need answers to the following questions if the information does not emerge without prompting: when did you last drink any alcohol? Do you drink daily or binge drink (have months alcohol-free)? What type of alcohol do you drink (spirits, beer)? How much do you drink each week now, and how much in the past? (Figure 22 allows you to calculate the number of units.) Have you ever been told you have an alcohol problem and told to stop drinking?

The CAGE questionnaire can be a useful aide-memoire for confirming suspicion of alcohol excess, particularly if the patient denies having an alcohol problem. With respect to drinking ask the patient if he or she has ever:

- **C** felt a need to *C*ut down?
- **A** been *A*nnoyed at the suggestion of a drinking problem?
- **G** felt *G*uilty about your drinking?
- **E** had to have a drink (*E*ye opener) in the morning?

Relevant past medical and surgical history

The details given here state that the patient has had a cholecystectomy, but it is always relevant to ask jaundiced patients if they are known to have gallstones. Patients can still have retained stones in the CBD despite cholecystectomy, as well as forming new stones *in situ*, and jaundice can develop as a result of inadvertent biliary or vascular complications following cholecystectomy.

Choledocholithiasis may present some time after previous cholecystectomy for gallstones: this may be due to silent stones having been missed in the CBD at the time of operation, or possibly formation of new stones *in situ*.

Drug history

It is essential to determine details of all prescribed and non-prescribed medications used by the patient in the 6 weeks before jaundice developed. Apparently innocent medications can cause drug-induced hepatotoxicity, common culprits including Augmentin (co-amoxiclav) and ibuprofen. Herbal and Chinese medications have also been implicated.

Travel history

Travel is a risk factor for jaundice: it is essential to know if patients have been abroad to a country where hepatitis A or hepatitis E is endemic, also if they have they been in contact with anyone else with viral hepatitis.

Other causes of liver disease

It is important and appropriate to take a sensitive history relating to previous intravenous drug abuse and a thorough sexual history. It is also relevant to enquire about a family

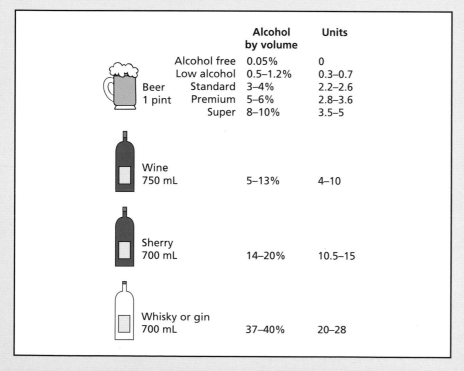

		Alcohol by volume	Units
	Alcohol free	0.05%	0
	Low alcohol	0.5–1.2%	0.3–0.7
Beer 1 pint	Standard	3–4%	2.2–2.6
	Premium	5–6%	2.8–3.6
	Super	8–10%	3.5–5
Wine 750 mL		5–13%	4–10
Sherry 700 mL		14–20%	10.5–15
Whisky or gin 700 mL		37–40%	20–28

▲**Fig. 22** Number of units of alcohol present in various alcoholic beverages (10 g of alcohol = 1 unit).

history of liver disease. Previous blood transfusions, a history of childhood jaundice or a history of pregnancy-associated jaundice occasionally give contributory information.

Is the patient developing hepatic encephalopathy?

A history of any change in the ability to concentrate, eg read the newspaper or do the crossword, can suggest early hepatic encephalopathy, as can reversal in the sleep–wake cycle with daytime sleepiness.

Examination

General features

As always when dealing with an acute case, the first priority is to decide if the patient is well, ill, very ill or nearly dead, and to begin resuscitation and get help from the intensive care unit immediately if required (as described in Sections 1.4.1 and 1.4.3). Then, in a patient presenting with jaundice, consider the diagnoses listed in Tables 23 and 24 and look for evidence of:

- sepsis (fever, tachycardia, hypotension, confusion);

- malignancy (cachexia, lymphadenopathy);

- chronic liver disease (see Section 1.2.2);

- alcohol withdrawal (agitation, hallucinations, tremor);

- hepatic encephalopathy (see Section 1.4.6);

- Wernicke's encephalopathy (nystagmus, ophthalmoplegia).

Abdomen

Look in particular for evidence of the following.

- Scars: previous cholecystectomy, previous resection of colorectal malignancy, previous surgery for

pancreatitis or pancreatic carcinoma.

- Liver: usually firm, tender and enlarged up to 10 cm in acute alcoholic hepatitis; may be irregular if there is associated cirrhosis, but firm irregular hepatomegaly must raise suspicion of malignancy (primary or secondary). A hepatic bruit may be heard in severe alcoholic hepatitis as well as with hepatocellular carcinoma.

- Splenomegaly: suggests portal hypertension in this context.

- Gallbladder: if palpable, remember Courvoisier's law, which states that in the presence of jaundice an enlarged gallbladder is unlikely to be due to gallstones (carcinoma of the pancreas or the lower biliary tree are more likely).

- Ascites: suggests chronic liver disease or malignancy.

- Melaena: indicates upper gastrointestinal bleeding.

Investigation

Routine blood tests and CXR

Check FBC, electrolytes, renal/liver/bone profiles, clotting screen, blood cultures, group and save. The pattern of abnormality on liver function tests is used to distinguish between a hepatitic process (raised alanine transaminase, ALT) and an obstructive biliary process (raised alkaline phosphatase, ALP), although distinction on these grounds is not infallible. The CXR may show evidence of lung cancer or metastatic disease.

⚠️ Gallstones can present acutely with ALT higher than ALP, and in end-stage liver disease liver enzymes can be normal.

Ultrasound examination of the abdomen

The key imaging test is ultrasound examination of the abdomen to help differentiate between hepatic and biliary causes of jaundice, and to provide evidence of chronic liver disease/portal hypertension.

- Liver, gallbladder and biliary tree: appearance of the liver parenchyma (fat infiltration, heterogeneous suggesting cirrhosis, focal lesion such as new hepatoma), intrahepatic and extrahepatic biliary ducts (dilation), gallbladder (stones, thick-walled suggesting inflammation), liver vasculature (portal vein thrombosis, hepatic vein abnormalities).

- Pancreas: not always well visualised, but is there a focal lesion?

- Spleen: enlargement suggests portal hypertension in this context; splenic varices may be seen.

- Ascites: consistent with portal hypertension or malignancy.

🔑 In the patient presenting with obstructive jaundice, consider the following:

- Gallstones.
- Pancreatic carcinoma/cholangiocarcinoma: usually painless.
- Pancreatitis: oedema/swelling of the pancreatic head can compress the bile duct.
- Budd–Chiari syndrome: acute hepatic vein obstruction results in painful hepatomegaly, ascites and jaundice (usually mild).

Further blood tests

These will be dictated by clinical suspicion and by the results of the routine investigations described above. If an acute infective hepatitis is thought most likely, then testing for hepatitis A, B and E, cytomegalovirus and Epstein–Barr virus will be appropriate. If it is thought that the patient has chronic liver disease, then investigation should be pursued as described in Section 1.1.7.

Further imaging

If there is a focal lesion in the liver or pancreas, then an abdominal CT scan should usually be the next investigation. In contrast, if ultrasonography suggests biliary pathology, then either endoscopic retrograde cholangiopancreatography (ERCP) (Fig. 23) or magnetic resonance cholangiopancreatography (MRCP) (Fig. 24) is indicated. In centres where both of these tests are available, ERCP should only be performed if it is likely that a therapeutic procedure is likely to be performed because of the associated morbidity and mortality.

Tissue biopsy

Broad indications for a liver biopsy are when the aetiology of liver disease is unclear, where the degree of liver damage determines the treatment (eg hepatitis B or C, autoimmune hepatitis) or where the nature of a focal lesion is unclear.

> ⚠️ Liver biopsy carries a significant risk of bleeding: the British Society of Gastroenterology suggests transjugular liver biopsy if the platelet count is $<40 \times 10^9$/L and/or the prothrombin time is prolonged by more than 6 seconds.

Management

If the patient is very ill, then resuscitate as described in Section 1.4.1. Specific management will depend on the diagnosis.

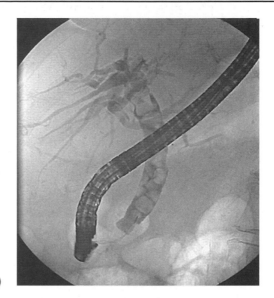

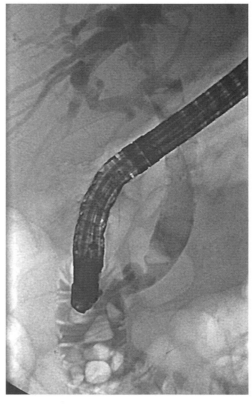

▲**Fig. 23** (a) Cholangiogram showing the CBD packed with stones. (b) The stones are seen within the duodenum following a sphincterotomy and trawling of the CBD with a balloon.

Cholangitis

> 🔑 Urgent drainage of the biliary system is required in acute ascending cholangitis with obstruction.

If the patient has high fever, rigors or is obviously septicaemic, then treat for septicaemia with the working diagnosis of ascending cholangitis. Most commonly gut organisms are the culprits, eg *Escherichia coli*, *Klebsiella* and

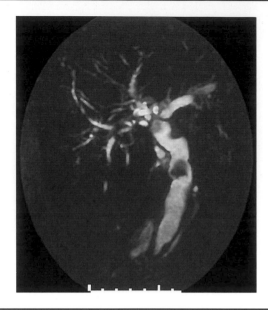

▲**Fig. 24** Magnetic resonance cholangiogram showing a stone in the CBD.

> ⚠ Accumulation of sedatives occurs in the presence of alcoholic hepatitis and/or cirrhosis and there is a risk of precipitating encephalopathy: review dosing on a daily basis and stop if the patient becomes drowsy.

> ⚠ Have a very low threshold for administering intravenous thiamine to any patient at risk of thiamine deficiency: the consequence of untreated or unrecognised Wernicke's encephalopathy are very serious.

Enterobacter species, enterococci and group D streptococci. Antibiotics with broad-spectrum cover should be given in accord with local antimicrobial guidelines, but these would typically comprise a third-generation cephalosporin, a quinolone such as ciprofloxacin or an antipseudomonal penicillin such as piperacillin/tazobactam (Tazocin).

The patient with an obstructed infected biliary tree will not get better until the obstruction is relieved. Insertion of a stent allows drainage around stones and can produce temporary clinical improvement in the ill patient with deranged clotting. Alternatively, sphincterotomy and stone extraction may be achieved at initial endoscopy (Fig. 23). Cholecystectomy is usual at a later date to remove the focus, unless comorbidity/frailty dictates otherwise.

The alcoholic with jaundice

The patient with jaundice in the context of alcoholic liver disease can be difficult to manage. If the patient deteriorates in hospital, the prognosis is poor. Progressive liver failure may develop with rising prothrombin time, increasing jaundice, encephalopathy, gastrointestinal haemorrhage (varices or gastropathy) and hepatorenal failure despite abstinence and good supportive medical care. Early active treatment is essential, as is early referral to a hepatologist.

Important aspects of treatment include assessment of prognosis based on clinical presentation and previous history of alcohol use, careful attention to fluid balance, scrupulous diagnosis and treatment of infection, aggressive nutrition, and prevention of alcohol withdrawal. Corticosteroids are used by some in the treatment of alcoholic hepatitis, but the timing and selection of patients who should receive these are controversial. UK liver centres do not offer liver transplantation for acute alcoholic hepatitis and those with chronic decompensated alcoholic liver disease need to demonstrate 6 months' abstinence and a commitment to lifelong alcohol avoidance.

1.4.6 Acute liver failure

Scenario

A 23-year-old woman is brought to the Emergency Department by her parents with agitation and confusion. After returning from a weekend away they found her at home with a suicide note and six empty packets of paracetamol by her side. On examination she is dehydrated, agitated, confused and has a tender liver edge.

Introduction

Acute liver failure is characterised by rapid deterioration of liver function resulting in altered mentation and coagulopathy in previously normal individuals: the simplest definition requires evidence of coagulopathy, usually an INR >1.5, and any degree of encephalopathy in a patient without pre-existing cirrhosis and with an illness of <26 weeks' duration. It is most commonly caused by paracetamol overdose, other drug-induced liver injury or viral hepatitis, but in 20% of cases the

TABLE 25 DIFFERENTIAL DIAGNOSIS OF ACUTE LIVER FAILURE

Common	Less common	Rare
Paracetamol (acetaminophen) overdose Drug or toxin induced[1] Cryptogenic (cause unknown)	Hepatitis A/hepatitis E Hepatitis B[2] Wilson's disease[2] Autoimmune chronic active hepatitis[2]	Hypotension/shock Venous outflow obstruction Hepatic veins (Budd–Chiari syndrome) Hepatic venules (veno-occlusive disease) Weil's disease (leptospirosis) Halothane Acute fatty liver of pregnancy

1. Including NSAIDs, ecstasy (methylenedioxymethamfetamine, MDMA), herbal remedies, mushroom poisoning, food contaminated with *Bacillus cereus* emetic toxin.
2. Patients with Wilson's disease, vertically acquired HBV or autoimmune hepatitis may be included despite the possibility of cirrhosis if their disease has only been recognised for <26 weeks.

cause remains unknown (Table 25). Overall short-term survival with liver transplantation is greater than 65%.

> ⚠ Acute liver failure is rare and carries a high mortality: early recognition, early and aggressive fluid resuscitation, and early liaison with a specialist liver unit improves outcomes.

History of the presenting problem

If severe encephalopathy is present the patient will not be able to give a reliable history, and information, if any is available, will have to come entirely from family or friends. In this case the diagnosis and cause of the problem seem reasonably clear-cut, but this will not always be so and it is necessary to determine if the presenting problem is acute liver

failure, if so what the likely cause is, and whether there is a background of chronic liver disease.

Is the problem acute liver failure?

The differential diagnosis of confusion/impaired consciousness is wide (Tables 26 and 27), so for fuller discussion of the clinical approach to the patient presenting with these problems see various clinical scenarios in *Acute Medicine* and *Medicine for the Elderly*. Further discussion here will be limited to the patient with acute liver failure.

Cause of acute liver failure

Has there been exposure to viral infection, drugs or other toxins? In this case the circumstances strongly suggest paracetamol overdose, but it is always appropriate to explore the following: is there any possibility the patient may have taken paracetamol, and if so how much and over how long a period? Has the patient recently been suicidal? Any previous overdoses?

Consider the other diagnoses listed in Table 25: is the patient at risk of any of these? A full drug history is required. What medications (prescribed and over-the-counter) have been taken in the last few weeks? Is the patient at risk of viral hepatitis? Has she travelled overseas recently?

TABLE 26 DIFFERENTIAL DIAGNOSIS OF CONFUSION

Frequency[1]	Condition
Common	Hypoglycaemia Urinary or chest infection Drug side effect/drug withdrawal Alcohol/alcohol withdrawal Post ictal Stroke Unreported discomfort, eg urinary retention Any cause of circulatory shock Any cause of hypoxia
Less common/rare	Electrolyte disturbance: hyponatraemia, hypercalcaemia Thiamine deficiency (Wernicke's encephalopathy) Other cerebral causes: metastases, haemorrhage (various), head injury[2] (concussion) Organ failure: hepatic encephalopathy, renal failure Other infective: meningitis, malaria Other endocrine: hyperthyroidism, hypothyroidism

1. Frequency refers to UK practice.
2. Head injury usually obvious, but not always.

> ⚠ Occasionally paracetamol overdose can occur unintentionally, with the drug taken over several days for medicinal purposes. Liver damage due to paracetamol is potentiated by concomitant alcoholic liver disease, malnutrition and some regular medications, eg phenytoin. Always take a very careful history of drug use.

TABLE 27 DIFFERENTIAL DIAGNOSIS OF COMA

Frequency[1]	Condition
Common	Hypoglycaemia
	Opioid toxicity
	Head injury[2]
	Post ictal
	Subarachnoid haemorrhage
	Stroke
	Alcohol
Less common/rare	Other poisoning: benzodiazepine, tricyclic antidepressant, carbon monoxide
	Other intracranial haemorrhage: extradural, subdural
	Hypothermia
	Electrolyte disturbance: hyponatraemia
	Organ failure: hepatic encephalopathy, advanced renal failure
	Infective: encephalitis, meningitis, malaria
	Non-convulsive status

1. Frequency refers to UK practice.
2. Head injury usually obvious, but not always.

Acute liver failure: other important questions

- Visual hallucinations: if these are associated with confusion, consider alcohol withdrawal in the differential diagnosis.

- Epileptic fits: these usually reflect alcohol withdrawal or focal cerebral disease, but seizures can occur at any stage of encephalopathy, and unrecognised hypoglycaemia must be excluded.

- Onset of confusion in relation to any history of jaundice: hepatic encephalopathy usually follows jaundice, and the time from onset of jaundice to encephalopathy is of prognostic significance. In paracetamol hepatotoxicity, encephalopathy typically occurs within 24–48 hours of jaundice and within 48–96 hours of the overdose.

- Abdominal pain: acute liver failure rarely causes pain, but there may be mild right-sided abdominal discomfort. If pain is prominent, consider hepatic vein occlusion (Budd–Chiari syndrome). In paracetamol overdose the pain typically subsides as the patient gets better.

Differential diagnosis of the patient with acute liver failure: important issues in the history

- Drug hepatotoxicity: exposure to any new drug, particularly an NSAID, in the 2 weeks preceding onset of jaundice; remember that it is important to exclude non-proprietary drugs such as herbal remedies.
- Viral hepatitis: risk factors for exposure to hepatitis B, eg in prostitutes, homosexuals, intravenous drug abusers and with use of potentially infected blood products from abroad.
- Wilson's disease: if less than 40 years old; there may be a family history and/or chronic neurological symptoms, eg tremor, change in handwriting.
- Autoimmune chronic active hepatitis: must always be excluded, particularly in middle-aged women; look for a previous medical history or family history of other autoimmune conditions, eg thyroid disease, rheumatoid arthritis.
- Leptospirosis (Weil's disease): if occupational or recreational exposure to stagnant water; look for myalgia and red eyes.
- Heart failure/ischaemic hepatitis: can mimic acute liver failure; when a patient develops acute liver failure in hospital, always look carefully in the medical and nursing records for documented periods of hypotension prior to presentation.
- Malignant infiltration of the liver by cancer or lymphoma: can occasionally present as acute liver failure.

Chronic liver disease

Is there a history of chronic confusion and/or poor concentration? This does not occur in acute liver failure and suggests chronic liver disease in this context. Has the patient got chronic liver disease or is she at risk of this (see Section 1.1.7)?

Other relevant history

Patients with acute liver failure may eventually need super-urgent liver transplantation. Particularly in paracetamol overdose it is useful to gather as much history as possible from relatives, friends and the patient's own GP about previous health and contact with the medical profession.

Examination

General features

If the patient is nearly dead (unrecordable BP, thready pulse, depressed conscious level), call immediately for help from the intensive care unit.

- Check vital signs: look in particular for evidence of volume depletion (cool peripheries, tachycardia, hypotension/postural hypotension, low JVP). Check pulse oximetry. In the early stages of acute hepatic failure vital signs are normal; late features include tachycardia and hypotension. A rising BP and a falling pulse rate are very late signs that indicate cerebral oedema and are associated with a poor prognosis.

> If the patient is peripherally shut down and hypotensive, insert two large-bore cannulae and start resuscitation immediately whilst completing the history and examination.

- Check Glasgow Coma Scale (GCS) score/grade hepatic encephalopathy: this is the hallmark of fulminant hepatic failure and comprises a spectrum of neuropsychiatric abnormalities in patients with liver dysfunction in the absence of other known brain disease. There are characteristic personality changes, intellectual impairment and a depressed level of consciousness. Note that focal neurological signs are not expected and their presence should alert to the possibility of a focal cerebral lesion, with intracerebral haemorrhage likely in this context. Decorticate/decerebrate posture and fixed pupils are late signs of irreversible cerebral oedema.

> **Grades of hepatic encephalopathy**
> - Grade I: altered mood, impaired concentration and psychomotor function.

> - Grade II: drowsy, inappropriate behaviour, able to talk.
> - Grade III: very drowsy, disorientated, agitated, aggressive.
> - Grade IV: coma, may respond to painful stimuli.

> ⚠ The onset of confusion or drowsiness in a patient with acute liver injury is ominous and necessitates advice from a liver unit.

- Stigmata of chronic liver disease (see Section 1.2.2): jaundice is often but not always seen at presentation with acute liver failure. Look for clues to risk behaviour, eg tattoos, injection sites, previous evidence of self-harm. If the patient is less than 40 years old, consider an ophthalmic slit lamp examination for Kayser–Fleischer rings of Wilson's disease.

- Look for signs of masquerading non-hepatic illnesses such as sepsis, heart failure and disseminated malignancy.

> Development of bilateral subconjunctival haemorrhages seems to be a feature peculiar to paracetamol-associated liver failure and should raise suspicion of this diagnosis in patients presenting late.

Abdomen

Right upper quadrant tenderness may be present. If the liver cannot be palpated, or the normal hepatic dullness cannot be detected by percussion, this may be indicative of decreased liver volume due to massive hepatocyte loss. An enlarged liver may be seen early in viral hepatitis or with malignant infiltration, congestive heart failure or acute Budd–Chiari syndrome.

Note that ascites would be very unusual in paracetamol poisoning but may occur with more gradual onset of acute hepatic insufficiency, ie so-called subacute liver failure.

Investigation

Routine tests in any very ill patient

- FBC, clotting screen/INR, electrolytes, glucose, renal/liver/bone function tests, magnesium, amylase/lipase, C-reactive protein (CRP), blood group and save.

- Blood, urine and sputum cultures.

- Arterial blood gases and lactate.

- Pregnancy test (if appropriate).

In the context of the patient with acute liver failure, look particularly for evidence of synthetic failure (coagulopathy, hypoglycaemia) and concurrent renal and/or respiratory failure. Hyponatraemia is common. One-third of patients with acute liver failure have pancreatitis at autopsy. Note that marked elevations in CRP are not in keeping with fulminant liver failure; if found, consider the possibility of sepsis as the primary illness and remember that this is a leading cause of death in acute liver failure. In paracetamol overdose an arterial lactate concentration >3.5 mmol/L early (4 hours) after admission to a liver unit or >3.0 mmol/L after fluid resuscitation (12 hours after admission) identifies patients who are likely to die early and who would therefore potentially benefit from transplantation. There is a high mortality of fulminant hepatitis E in pregnant women.

> ⚠ The liver function tests themselves may aid in understanding the aetiology of the liver disease, but the transaminase level itself is of no prognostic significance and just indicates liver cell damage.

> 🔑 Where the prothrombin time (PT) in seconds is greater than the time after a paracetamol overdose (in hours), eg a PT of 40 seconds 30 hours after the overdose as opposed to a PT of 50 seconds 60 hours after the overdose, there is a particular risk of developing liver failure.

Blood tests to determine the cause of acute liver failure

These should clearly be determined by the clinical context. In some instances, such as the case described here, the diagnosis will be clear-cut and extensive investigation is not required to establish the cause of liver failure, but where the cause is not obvious the following would be appropriate.

- Paracetamol level.

- Toxicology screen as appropriate.

- Viral hepatitis serology: anti-HAV IgM, HBsAg, anti-HBc IgM, anti-HEV, anti-HCV (extended screen if these are negative and no other diagnosis established, including herpes simplex virus (HSV), cytomegalovirus (CMV), Epstein–Barr virus, adenovirus, parvovirus B19).

- Caeruloplasmin level (if patient <40 years).

- Autoimmune markers: antinuclear antibodies, liver antibodies, immunoglobulin levels.

- HIV status.

- Leptospiral serology.

> ⚠ Surface antigen is cleared from the serum by the time of presentation with jaundice in up to 5% of patients with fulminant hepatitis due to hepatitis B virus: diagnosis therefore rests on an appropriate pattern of antibody response (eg IgM anti-core) or DNA levels.

Abdominal imaging

Ultrasound is particularly useful to look for evidence of background chronic liver disease (splenomegaly, varices, ascites, portal vein thrombosis), and it is also the first-line investigation if Budd–Chiari syndrome is suspected. Cross-sectional imaging with CT should be performed if the patient is stable enough and the diagnosis is at all in doubt.

Management

Early involvement of specialist hepatology services is important in managing patients with acute liver failure. The key aspects of management include the following.

- Oxygenation: give high-flow oxygen to maintain arterial saturation >92%.

- Treat/prevent hypovolaemia: use 4.5% albumin (rather than 0.9% saline in this context).

- Treat/prevent hypoglycaemia: give 10% dextrose (or, if needed, and by a central line, 50% dextrose) at a rate to keep fingerprick blood glucose in the range 4–7 mmol/L.

- Correct electrolyte abnormalities, including phosphate: but note that hyponatraemia is due to water excess and not to sodium deficiency and should not be treated by infusion of saline.

- Monitor renal function closely: renal replacement therapy should be instituted sooner rather than later if the patient develops renal failure.

- Avoid unnecessary medications: in particular NSAIDs, diuretics, opiates and sedatives.

- Enteral or parenteral nutrition: should be initiated without delay.

- *N*-Acetylcysteine: give 150 mg/kg in 1 L 5% dextrose over 24 hours (note different regimen if given as a specific antidote to paracetamol toxicity; see below).

- Prophylaxis against sepsis: give broad-spectrum antibiotics and fluconazole.

- Prophylaxis against gastrointestinal stress ulceration, eg ranitidine or omeprazole.

- Consider treatments to minimise absorption of nitrogenous substances from the gut (not used in all liver centres): disaccharide laxative, eg lactulose, in dose sufficient to produce two to three soft stools daily; enemas; broad-spectrum poorly absorbed antibiotic, eg neomycin 1 g qds by mouth.

> ⚠ Avoid precipitating Wernicke's encephalopathy: if there is a history of high alcohol intake or malnourishment, give thiamine intravenously before giving glucose, eg Pabrinex (thiamine) intravenous high potency, 10 mL over 10 minutes three times daily.

> 🔑 Do not routinely correct coagulopathy: bleeding is rare in acute liver failure and the PT is an important prognostic indicator.

Hepatic encephalopathy

The patient's neurological status must be reviewed regularly: if hepatic encephalopathy develops, progression from grade I to grade IV and development of cerebral oedema may occur within an hour or two. Patients who are agitated or aggressive may need ventilation to enable care to be given; those with grade III or IV encephalopathy should be ventilated electively because of the risk of cerebral oedema; and those with grade II encephalopathy should be considered for ventilation to facilitate safe transfer to a liver unit.

Cerebral oedema is not likely in patients with grade I–II encephalopathy, but with progression to grade III the risk increases to 25–35% and with grade IV coma to 65–75% or more. The signs of hypertension, bradycardia and irregular respirations (Cushing's triad) are not uniformly present; these and other neurological changes such as pupillary dilatation or signs of decerebration are typically evident only late in the course. Liver units vary in their monitoring for, and management of, this condition, but many will directly measure cerebral perfusion pressure (CPP) and intracranial pressure (ICP), maintaining ICP below 20–25 mmHg and CPP above 50–60 mmHg if possible. Strategies for care include nursing at 20–30°, hyperventilation to reduce CO_2, controlled hypothermia, mannitol boluses (0.5–1 g/kg repeated as long as serum osmolality <320 mosmol/L), controlled hypernatraemia (boluses of 30% hypertonic saline to maintain serum sodium 145–155 mmol/L), and occasionally short-acting barbiturates such as thiopental.

Specific treatments

Paracetamol overdose Liver failure from paracetamol overdose is preventable if the patient presents early and *N*-acetylcysteine is correctly administered, and this treatment improves prognosis even in those who present over 16 hours afterwards. Following loading

TABLE 28 GUIDELINES FOR REFERRAL TO SPECIALIST CENTRES IN CASES OF PARACETAMOL TOXICITY ACCORDING TO FINDINGS ON DAYS 2–4 FOLLOWING THE OVERDOSE		
Day 2 (24–48 hours)	**Day 3 (48–72 hours)**	**Day 4 (72–96 hours)**
Arterial pH <7.3 INR >3 Encephalopathy Creatinine >200 µmol/L Hypoglycaemia	Arterial pH <7.3 INR >4.5 Encephalopathy Creatinine >200 µmol/L	Any rise in INR Encephalopathy Creatinine >250 µmol/L

(150 mg/kg iv over 15 minutes followed by 50 mg/kg over 4 hours) continue maintenance dose of 150 mg/kg for 24 hours, which can be given as a concentrated solution if there is a problem with fluid overload. If appropriate refer the patient to a specialist centre (Table 28).

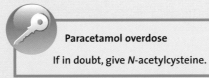

Paracetamol overdose

If in doubt, give *N*-acetylcysteine.

Other causes of acute liver failure
Other specific therapies will depend on the particular diagnosis, eg prednisolone in autoimmune hepatitis, lamivudine in hepatitis B, aciclovir in HSV or varicella infection, ganciclovir in CMV infection, delivery in pregnancy-associated disease. Clearly such management needs to be carefully discussed with a hepatologist.

Further comments

Criteria for liver transplantation
Urgent hepatic transplantation is indicated in acute liver failure where

prognostic indicators suggest a high likelihood of death. Classically, those listed for 'super-urgent' liver transplantation are predicted to have a survival of less than 3 days without a new organ. The King's College Criteria recommend transplantation in the following circumstances.

- Paracetamol-induced acute liver failure: arterial pH <7.3 following adequate volume resuscitation (irrespective of coma grade) *or* PT >100 seconds (INR >6.5) and serum creatinine >300 µmol/L in patients in grade III/IV coma.

- Non-paracetamol-induced acute liver failure: PT >100 seconds (irrespective of coma grade) *or* any three of the following (irrespective of coma grade): drug toxicity/indeterminate cause of acute liver failure; age <10 years or >40 years; jaundice to coma interval >7 days; PT >50 seconds (INR >3.5); serum bilirubin >300 µmol/L.

Amendments continue to be suggested and prognostic markers such as lactate, alpha-fetoprotein, phosphate and factor V levels have been used by some.

2.1 Oesophageal disease

2.1.1 Gastro-oesophageal reflux disease

Aetiology/pathophysiology/ pathology

Reflux of gastric acid into the lower oesophagus can cause mucosal injury (reflux oesophagitis). Chronic reflux oesophagitis may induce the appearance of ectopic gastric and intestinal mucosa in the lower oesophagus (gastric or intestinal metaplasia), a change termed 'Barrett's oesophagus' that is considered premalignant because it is associated with an increased risk of oesophageal adenocarcinoma. Chronic reflux oesophagitis may also lead to fibrotic healing and the formation of a peptic stricture.

Incompetence of the lower oesophageal sphincter is the main factor in reflux of acid. Gastric acid secretion is usually normal. Hiatal hernias, occurring in 10–15% of the general population, are more prevalent with increasing severity of reflux disease and may contribute to abnormal reflux by both reducing basal lower oesophageal pressure and impairing effective oesophageal clearance of acid (Fig. 25).

Reflux may result in a spectrum of damage to the oesophagus, ranging from microscopic changes only through to circumferential

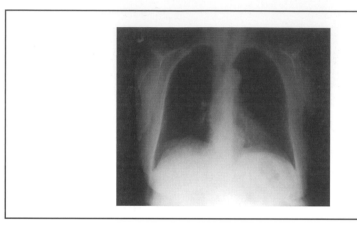

▲**Fig. 25** CXR showing a hiatus hernia behind the heart.

oesophagitis with ulceration and stricture formation. This can be graded using the Savary–Miller classification.

- Grade I: one or more non-confluent erosions.

- Grade II: confluent but not circumferential erosions.

- Grade III: circumferential erosive oesophagitis.

- Grade IV: grade III plus ulceration, stricture formation or Barrett's oesophagus.

Epidemiology

Gastro-oesophageal reflux symptoms (retrosternal burning, acid regurgitation) are common and occur on a daily basis in up to 10% of the population. Only about one-third of patients will have endoscopic evidence of oesophagitis. Peptic strictures occur in 7–23% of patients with untreated reflux oesophagitis.

Clinical presentation

Common

Burning retrosternal pain aggravated by lying down or bending forwards, and by spicy foods, citrus fruits and alcohol. Regurgitation of acid, water brash, chest pain, odynophagia (painful swallowing) and dysphagia.

> Oesophagitis and Barrett's oesophagus can be entirely asymptomatic. Conversely, reflux symptoms can be severe without endoscopic or histological evidence of oesophagitis.

Uncommon

Haematemesis or iron-deficiency anaemia.

Physical signs

Usually no physical signs. Occasionally, severe acid reflux into the pharynx can lead to hoarseness and pharyngitis. Weight loss if there has been a delayed presentation of an oesophageal stricture.

Investigation/staging

Upper gastrointestinal endoscopy
Indicated if troublesome or refractory reflux symptoms.

> ⚠ • Gastroscopy is mandatory in those who have alarm symptoms (haematemesis, dysphasia, weight loss, anaemia) and desirable in middle-aged or elderly patients with new onset of symptoms.
> • Patients in their twenties or early thirties who require infrequent, intermittent courses of acid-suppressing therapy probably do not warrant endoscopy, but those with persistent symptoms requiring long-term therapy should be examined to define the extent and severity of oesophagitis (or presence of Barrett's oesophagus) and thereby guide therapy.

Oesophageal manometry and 24-hour ambulatory pH monitoring
This is useful in patients with atypical symptoms, in those who do not respond to acid-suppressant therapy, and as part of the work-up for patients considered for antireflux surgery (along with oesophageal manometry).

Differential diagnosis
Common differential diagnoses include the following.

- Cardiac pain.

- Oesophageal carcinoma: benign-looking peptic strictures must be brushed and biopsied to exclude malignancy.

- Infections with herpes simplex or *Candida*.

- Drugs (eg alendronate, NSAIDs, ferrous sulphate, potassium salts) that may cause oesophagitis.

- Radiotherapy-induced oesophagitis (eg treatment of bronchial carcinoma).

Treatment

Emergency
Patients with dysphagia need rapid assessment with either a barium or Gastrograffin swallow followed by endoscopy. Barium swallow is usually performed first to define the position and extent of any stricture. Patients with a stricture demonstrated on barium swallow should proceed to endoscopy for biopsy and brushings to exclude malignancy. All patients with benign peptic oesophageal strictures should be commenced on a proton pump inhibitor (PPI) to prevent further acid reflux and damage. Concurrent oesophagitis *per se* may contribute to the dysphagia. If symptoms are significant, oesophageal dilatation should be performed. Initial improvement occurs in >80%, although one-third require repeat dilatation within 12 months despite acid-suppression therapy.

Short-term
Treatment of uncomplicated gastro-oesophageal reflux should be directed at alleviating the symptoms. A graded approach is usual, starting with antacids and lifestyle measures (stopping smoking, avoiding precipitants), then histamine H_2 receptor antagonists with or without prokinetic agents (eg metoclopramide), and finally PPIs or antireflux surgery. When oesophagitis is demonstrated endoscopically or microscopically, aggressive initial treatment with a PPI, followed by an H_2 receptor antagonist, and eventually symptomatic treatment with antacids should be initiated. Healing of oesophagitis (grade II or more severe) is desirable to prevent

complications such as stricture formation or Barrett's metaplasia.

Long-term
Many patients with symptomatic gastro-oesophageal reflux relapse following cessation of medical therapy. PPIs are the most effective agents in the initial healing of reflux oesophagitis (80–90% within 8 weeks with standard doses) and in subsequent maintenance therapy. Aggressive acid-suppression therapy with PPIs has been shown to decrease the need for repeat dilatation of oesophageal peptic strictures.

Complications

Common
Most patients with gastro oesophageal reflux disease can be well controlled with acid-suppression therapy. Relapse of symptoms is common on withdrawal of treatment. It is estimated that up to one-quarter of patients with untreated reflux oesophagitis will develop strictures. Long-term acid reflux is important in the development of Barrett's oesophagus.

Prognosis
The advent of the powerful PPI agents means the vast majority of patients can be rendered asymptomatic. Antireflux surgery is an alternative where medical therapy fails, or if the patient is young and unwilling to take medications indefinitely. Although reflux disease has little effect on life expectancy, it may predispose to the development of oesophageal adenocarcinoma. Long-term severe reflux predisposes to Barrett's oesophagus with its malignant potential.

Prevention
Aggressive control of acid secretion is likely to be important

in preventing peptic stricture formation in those with significant reflux oesophagitis. Once a stricture has formed, long-term therapy with a PPI is indicated.

Disease associations

Scleroderma may result in severe oesophagitis and stricture formation.

FURTHER READING

Katz PO, ed. Gastroesophageal reflux disease. *Gastroenterol. Clin. North Am.* 1999; 28.

Vigneri S, Termini R, Leandro G, *et al.* A comparison of five maintenance therapies for reflux esophagitis. *N. Engl. J. Med.* 1995; 333: 1106–10.

Wu AH, Tseng CC and Bernstein L. Hiatal hernia, reflux symptoms, body size, and risk of esophageal and gastric adenocarcinoma. *Cancer* 2003; 98: 940–8.

2.1.2 Achalasia and oesophageal dysmotility

Aetiology/pathophysiology/ pathology

The cause of disordered oesphageal motility is generally unknown. Achalasia is the most severe form, characterised by a hypertensive lower oesophageal sphincter (LOS) with failure of LOS relaxation in response to swallowing. Peristalsis is absent in the body of the oesophagus, which becomes progressively dilated. Histological examination reveals loss of myenteric plexus ganglia.

Epidemiology

Achalasia is rare, with an approximate incidence of 1 in 100,000 in the West. Less severe forms of oesophageal dysmotility may be more widespread and may account for some cases of apparent gastro-oesophageal reflux disease without documented acid reflux or response to acid-suppressive treatment.

Clinical presentation

Common

Dysphagia (difficulty in swallowing) and odynophagia (painful swallowing) are typical. Regurgitation may cause nocturnal cough and respiratory complications in achalasia.

Physical signs

Often absent, but weight loss may be evident.

Investigation/staging

Barium or Gastrograffin swallow

This should be performed before endoscopy, showing food debris in the oesophagus with dilatation in later stages and a smooth, tapered 'bird's beak' at the distal end (Fig. 26).

> Gastroscopy should always be performed to exclude malignancy at the gastro-oesophageal junction: this can mimic achalasia, particularly in elderly people.

Manometry

The typical pattern of progressive peristaltic contraction waves in the oesophagus in response to swallowing is lost. There may be diffuse spasm (diffuse oesophageal spasm) or intense prolonged contractions ('nutcracker' oesophagus). In achalasia the body of the oesophagus fails to contract peristaltically and there is increased pressure at the LOS, which fails to relax in response to swallowing.

Differential diagnosis

The pain associated with oesophageal dysmotility may mimic cardiac or pleuritic chest pain. Chagas' disease, caused by South American trypanosomal infection, is rare but may present with identical clinical, endoscopic and radiological features to achalasia.

Treatment

Medical

Explanation and reassurance are essential. Prokinetic agents such as metoclopramide may provide some symptomatic relief. Calcium antagonists (eg nifedipine 10 mg tds) or nitrates (eg isosorbide) can be tried, but response is variable. It is pragmatic to offer a proton pump inhibitor to minimise any effect of gastro-oesophageal reflux. Endoscopic and surgical treatments should be explored if achalasia progresses to cause dysphagia and regurgitation.

Pneumatic (balloon) dilatation or surgical myotomy (Heller's)

Results are comparable, with 75–85% having excellent relief of their symptoms. Perforation occurs in 1–5% after dilatation. Late stricture formation occurs in about 3% of surgically treated patients.

Intrasphincteric injection of botulinum toxin

This is as effective as pneumatic dilatation at 4 weeks but not at 6 months, when repeat injection is often required.

Complications

Common

- Risk of oesophageal carcinoma is increased about 15-fold in patients with achalasia.

- Reflux oesophagitis and stricture formation (<1%) may occur after pneumatic dilatation.

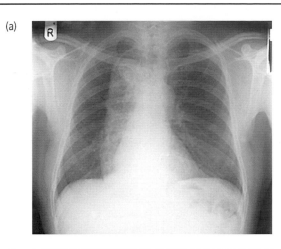

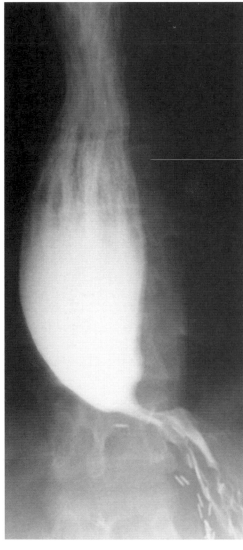

▲ **Fig. 26** (a) CXR of achalasia: note the widened mediastinum due to the grossly distended oesophagus. (b) Barium swallow of achalasia: the distal end of the dilated oesophagus has a characteristic 'beaked' appearance.

Prognosis

Over 90% of patients with achalasia are improved following pneumatic dilatation or surgical myotomy. Repeat dilatation is frequently required.

FURTHER READING

Leyden JE, Moss AC and MacMathuna P. Endoscopic pneumatic dilation versus botulinum toxin injection in the management of primary achalasia. *Cochrane Database Syst Rev* 2006; (4): CD005046.

– – – – – – – – – – – – – – – – – –

Seelig MH, DeVault KR, Seelig SK, *et al.* Treatment of achalasia: recent advances in surgery. *J. Clin. Gastroenterol.* 1999; 28: 202–7.

2.1.3 Oesophageal cancer and Barrett's oesophagus

Aetiology/pathophysiology/ pathology

Risk factors for carcinoma of oesophagus are shown in Table 29. Oesophageal carcinoma is microscopically squamous cell or adenocarcinoma.

Barrett's oesophagus is defined as replacement of the normal squamous epithelial lining of the oesophagus by metaplastic columnar epithelium. It is strongly associated with chronic gastro-oesophageal reflux of acid, which is thought to damage the normal lining with replacement by columnar, acid-resistant lining. The main importance of Barrett's oesophagus is that it is probably a precursor lesion of oesophageal adenocarcinoma, with a 40% lifetime risk of this complication in patients with a segment of Barrett's >3 cm long.

Epidemiology

Worldwide, squamous cell carcinoma is most common. There are geographical variations in its

TABLE 29 RISK FACTORS FOR CARCINOMA OF OESOPHAGUS

Squamous cell carcinoma	Adenocarcinoma
Smoking	Barrett's oesophagus
Alcohol	Gastro-oesphageal reflux
Malnutrition	
Achalasia	
Postcricoid web[1]	
Familial tylosis[2]	

1. Brown–Kelly–Paterson/Plummer–Vinson syndrome.
2. Hyperkeratosis of palms of hands and soles of feet.

incidence, with the highest rates (>100 per 100,000) in China, Iran and South Africa. In the Western world the incidence of adenocarcinoma of the oesophagus is rising rapidly for reasons that are unknown, and it is more common than squamous cell carcinoma.

The true prevalence of Barrett's oesophagus is unknown since many cases are silent and therefore not detected. About 10% of patients undergoing upper gastrointestinal endoscopy for reflux symptoms are found to have a columnar-lined oesophagus (Barrett's), and half will have specialised intestinal-type lining. Autopsy studies suggest a prevalence of around 1%.

Clinical presentation

Common
Progressive dysphagia with weight loss is the usual presentation of oesophageal cancer. Initially subjects may have dysphagia only for solids such as meat and bread, eventually reporting difficulty swallowing purees and liquids. May be discovered as part of the work-up of iron-deficiency anaemia.

Barrett's oesophagus may be asymptomatic, or it may be discovered as a result of diagnostic tests for gastro-oesophageal reflux symptoms.

Uncommon
- Dyspepsia or heartburn.
- Pain due to local invasion into the spine or intercostal nerves.
- Hoarseness due to involvement of the recurrent laryngeal nerve by middle and upper third oesophageal carcinomas.

Rare
- Tracheo-oesophageal fistulae.

Physical signs
Signs may reflect the extent and duration of disease, with weight loss, evidence of complications such as aspiration pneumonia, and rarely hoarseness due to tumour invasion of the recurrent laryngeal nerve.

Investigation/staging

Barium or Gastrograffin swallow
This is the initial investigation of choice for patients presenting with dysphagia (Fig. 27).

Upper gastrointestinal endoscopy
The key test for obtaining multiple biopsies for histology and brushings for cytology for a tissue diagnosis. In Barrett's, the oesophagus has a characteristic red, velvety, columnar epithelium extending proximally from the gastro-oesophageal junction (proximal end of gastric

rugal folds), with biopsy confirming columnar metaplasia (Fig. 28).

CT of the thorax and abdomen
Undertaken to look for evidence of local invasion into mediastinal structures and for hepatic or pulmonary metastases.

Endoscopic ultrasound
If available this provides more accurate local staging of the tumour. Unfortunately most are advanced at presentation: T3, with invasion through the oesophageal wall into the adventitia; or T4, with spread into adjacent structures, eg aorta, pulmonary vessels.

Differential diagnosis
- Benign oesophageal stricture: usually obvious at endoscopy, confirmed with biopsy and brushings, but repeat sampling if clinical suspicion but histology negative.
- Gastric carcinoma (usually from the cardia) invading the lower oesophagus.

Note that biopsy from a point distal to the squamous–columnar junction (eg from the proximal end of a hiatus hernia) will lead to a false-positive diagnosis of Barrett's oesophagus.

Treatment

Emergency
Presentation with complete or near-complete obstruction (liquids/liquidised food) is not unusual, in which case dilatation may be needed at the time of diagnostic endoscopy.

> ⚠ The risk of oesophageal perforation is higher with dilatation of malignant compared with benign strictures.

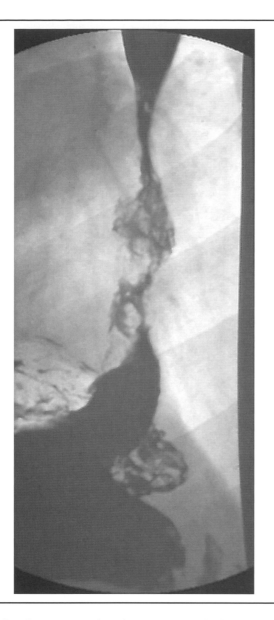

▲**Fig. 27** Barium swallow showing an irregular malignant stricture in the distal oesophagus.

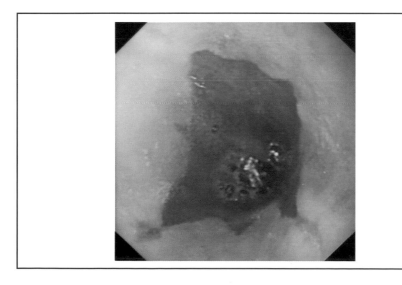

◄**Fig. 28** Barrett's oesophagus. The squamous–columnar junction lies above the gastro-oesophageal junction.

Short-term

Aim is rapid work-up to select appropriate candidates (less than one-third) for curative surgery, usually with thoracoabdominal CT and endoscopic ultrasound if available. Preoperative enteral or parenteral nutrition and physiotherapy are important. Subtotal oesophagectomy with anastomosis to fashioned gastric 'tube' is often employed.

Long-term

Palliation indicated in most cases, with either endoscopic or radiological positioning of expandable metal stents, laser photocoagulation or radiotherapy (internal or external).

Complications

Oesophagectomy

Anastomosis may leak or dehisce (has less rich blood supply compared with rest of intestine).

Oesophageal stent

Perforation during stent placement and laser photocoagulation. Stent migration.

Prognosis

Morbidity

Aim with the majority is palliation, ie ensuring reasonable swallowing.

Mortality

Overall median survival <1 year; 5-year survival rate 5%. Earlier stage and absence of lymph node involvement yields better results. There is 5–10% mortality with oesophagectomy.

Prevention

Primary

Aggressive suppression of acid secretion in patients with Barrett's oesophagus or reflux oesophagitis. Long-term acid suppression may arrest or reverse Barrett's changes.

Endoscopic surveillance for adenocarcinoma

This involves yearly endoscopy with multiple quadrantic biopsies, particularly if the segment of Barrett's is long (>3 cm) and shows intestinal-type metaplasia. Junctional and gastric-type metaplasia probably have very low malignant potential and are not usually surveyed.

Endoscopic ablative therapy

The role of laser, photodynamic therapy or electrocoagulation to ablate Barrett's oesophagus is unclear, but may be considered for those who have high-grade dysplasia or carcinoma *in situ* and whose comorbidity prevents surgery.

FURTHER READING

Allum WH, Griffin SM, Watson A and Colin-Jones D (on behalf of the Association of Upper Gastrointestinal Surgeons of Great Britain and Ireland, the British Society of Gastroenterology, and the British Association of Surgical Oncology). Guidelines for the management of oesophageal and gastric cancer. *Gut* 2002; 50 (Suppl. 5): v1–v23. Full text available at http://www.bsg.org.uk/

Enzinger PC and Mayer RJ. Esophageal cancer. *N. Engl. J. Med.* 2003; 349: 2241–52.

Spechler SJ. Clinical practice: Barrett's esophagus. *N. Engl. J. Med.* 2002; 346: 836–42.

Watson A, Heading RC and Shepherd NA, eds. *Guidelines for the Diagnosis and Management of Barrett's Columnar-lined Oesophagus*. London: British Society for Gastroenterology, 2005. Full text available at http://www.bsg.org.uk/

2.2 Gastric disease

2.2.1 Peptic ulceration and *Helicobacter pylori*

Aetiology/pathophysiology/ pathology

Helicobacter pylori infection and NSAID use are the two most common aetiological factors. Risk of peptic ulceration appears to be higher in NSAID users if they are also infected with *H. pylori*. There are different *H. pylori* strains, Cag-A being associated with more severe gastritis and intestinal metaplasia. *H. pylori* is unique in that it produces a urease that is made use of in diagnostic tests.

Epidemiology

In the UK, serological testing for *H. pylori* shows that up to 50% of 50 year olds and up to 20% of 20 year olds have been infected. This is a cohort effect and does not mean that 1% acquire the infection each year. *H. pylori* causes 90% of duodenal ulcers and 60% of gastric ulcers.

The lifetime risk of duodenal ulcer is 4–10% and of gastric ulcer 3–4%, males more than females.

Clinical presentation

Common

- Epigastric pain or indigestion.

- Lethargy from anaemia.

- Melaena and/or haematemesis.

Uncommon

If present in the pylorus there may be gastric outlet obstruction with vomiting.

Rare

Perforation with abdominal pain and signs of an acute abdomen.

Physical signs

- Anaemia.

- Epigastric tenderness.

Investigations/staging

Endoscopy

- To establish the diagnosis and to take biopsies from a gastric ulcer to ensure it is benign.

- Antral and gastric body biopsies for *H. pylori*.

- Risk of rebleeding can also be assessed in those presenting with haematemesis or melaena.

> Some gastric ulcers are malignant despite appearing benign endoscopically, hence biopsy is vital.

H. pylori detection

There are many methods by which *H. pylori* can be identified. Serological testing for IgA or IgG antibodies to *H. pylori* is only useful if previously untreated. Samples taken at endoscopy can be subjected to a CLO test or histological examination (silver stain) (Figs 29 and 30).

> Serology cannot be used to assess whether the infection has been successfully eradicated with treatment, as antibodies persist often for decades.

^{13}C urea breath test

A non-invasive method of assessing whether *H. pylori* has been successfully eradicated.

More novel methods of detecting *H. pylori* include measurement of bacterial antigens within stool samples.

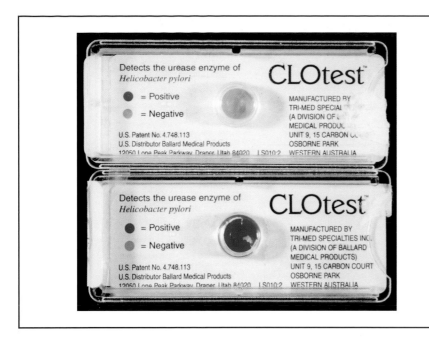

▲**Fig. 29** CLO test. This relies on the fact that *H. pylori* produces a urease. A gastric biopsy is placed on the test card. If *H. pylori* is present, the indicator turns from yellow to red. A result is obtained in 1 hour.

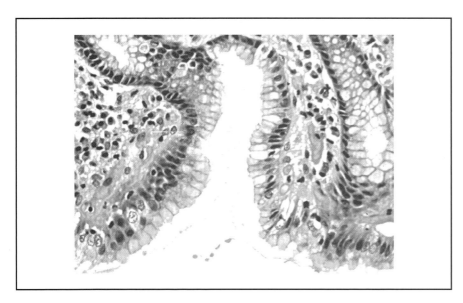

▲**Fig. 30** Histology of gastric mucosal biopsy showing the presence of *H. pylori* on the epithelial surface.

Differential diagnosis

- If abdominal pain, see Sections 1.1.6 and 1.4.4.

- If gastrointestinal haemorrhage, see Section 1.4.3.

Treatment

Emergency

See Section 1.4.3. Endoscopic therapy can be used to try to control bleeding using injection (adrenaline) and thermal contact devices (electrocoagulation).

Short-term

Eradication of H. pylori

Triple-drug regimens are effective in 80–95% of cases, eg 7 days of twice-daily proton pump inhibitor (PPI), clarithromycin 500 mg bd or amoxicillin 1 g bd, and metronidazole 500 mg bd.

Reinfection following eradication of *H. pylori* is rare in adults. Antibiotic resistance to metronidazole and/or clarithromycin occurs in 10–20%. Some patients require further triple-therapy regimens, which may require modification using culture and sensitivities from gastric aspiration.

Ulcer healing Six weeks of PPI to heal the ulcer.

Long-term

A patient who has had a complicated peptic ulcer (bleeding or perforation) should probably remain on long-term antisecretory therapy (PPI or histamine H_2 receptor blocker). If an NSAID is required following a gastrointestinal bleed, then a cyclooxygenase (COX)-2 inhibitor combined with a PPI has been suggested, although COX-2 inhibitors are not currently in favour. If NSAID therapy is required after an uncomplicated peptic ulcer, consider using misoprostol or a PPI in addition.

Complications

- Perforation and bleeding.

- Gastric carcinoma: less than 3% of gastric ulcers are malignant.

- Oesophageal reflux: there is concern that eradication of *H. pylori* may be associated with an increased incidence of oesophageal reflux.

Prognosis

Most peptic ulcers heal when a PPI is used, but 20% will develop recurrent ulceration even if *H. pylori* infection is eradicated.

Prevention

Primary

Avoidance of NSAIDs and smoking. Use misoprostol or PPI with an NSAID.

Disease associations

Gastrinoma is associated with multiple peptic ulcers. May occur in isolation or associated with multiple endocrine neoplasia (MEN) type 1.

FURTHER READING

Malfertheiner P, Megraud F, O'Morain C, *et al*. Current concepts in the management of *Helicobacter pylori* infection: the Maastricht III Consensus Report. *Gut* 2007; 56: 772–81.

- - - - - - - - - - - - - - - - - -

Rostom A, Dube C, Wells G, *et al*. Prevention of NSAID-induced gastroduodenal ulcers. *Cochrane Database Syst Rev* 2002; (4): CD002296.

2.2.2 Gastric carcinoma

Aetiology/pathophysiology/pathology

Gastric carcinomas are adenocarcinomas and can be classified histologically as diffuse or intestinal. They are associated with atrophic gastritis and intestinal metaplasia, but there is no evidence that long-term drug-induced achlorhydria is associated with gastric cancer. Distal gastrectomy is associated with a 12-fold increased risk of gastric cancer after 15–20 years. There is also increasing evidence of an association between *Helicobacter pylori* and gastric cancer, with prospective serological studies showing a three- to six-fold increased risk, mainly of distal tumours. Countries with high rates of gastric cancer also have a high incidence of *H. pylori* infection.

Epidemiology

The highest incidence is in Japan and China; in the USA, incidence is 10 per 100,000. Overall the incidence is falling, but adenocarcinoma affecting the cardia and gastro-oesophageal junction is becoming more common. It rarely occurs before the age of 40 years, peaking in the seventies.

Clinical presentation

Common

Small superficial tumours are often asymptomatic. Later symptoms are weight loss (61%), abdominal pain (51%), nausea (34%) and dysphagia (26%). Malaise due to iron-deficiency anaemia. Acute upper gastrointestinal haemorrhage.

Rare

Vomiting from pyloric obstruction.

Physical signs

Common

Usually there are no abnormal clinical findings.

Uncommon

- Epigastric mass.
- Malignant ascites due to peritoneal seeding.

Rare

Enlarged supraclavicular lymph node (Virchow's).

> The 'red flag' symptoms for urgent referral for suspected gastric cancer all suggest advanced disease; there are no symptoms of early gastric cancer.

Investigations

- FBC: an iron-deficiency anaemia is present in 42%.
- Tumour markers: carcinoembryonic antigen is not helpful diagnostically. It is elevated in 10–20% of patients with resectable tumour.
- Endoscopy: essential for histological diagnosis and assessment of size and position of the tumour (Fig. 31).

- Abdominal CT: used for staging to assess whether a tumour is surgically resectable. Staging is graded from I to IV, dependent on the TNM (tumour, nodes, metastases) classification.
- Endoscopic ultrasound: useful in the staging of gastric neoplasia as it gives information on depth of invasion locally as well as lymph node involvement and may identify tumours that can be removed endoscopically by endomucosal resection.

Treatment

Surgery

Indicated if early tumour confined to stomach (ie stage I).

Chemotherapy

Neoadjuvant chemotherapy may reduce tumour bulk and invasion prior to surgery. Combined surgery and chemotherapy are better than chemotherapy alone.

Conservative

Indicated for linitus plasticus (involving whole of stomach) or those with locally invasive and widespread metastatic disease.

Complications

Haemorrhage.

Prognosis

The 5-year overall survival rates are poor in the UK at 15%. Stage I (confined to stomach) with surgery has a 5-year survival rate of 50% in the UK and 90% in Japan.

Prevention

Screening by endoscopy is advocated in Japan, where 40–60% of early gastric cancers can be identified, but this is not the case in the UK, Europe and the USA.

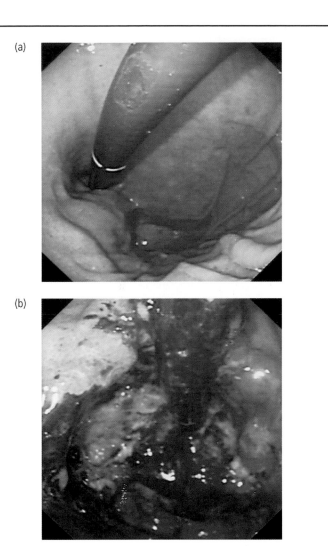

(a)

(b)

▲ **Fig. 31** Endoscopic appearance of (a) normal gastro-oesophageal junction and (b) gastric carcinoma.

Disease associations

Pernicious anaemia is associated with a two- to three-fold increased risk of carcinoma of stomach.

Cunningham D, Allum WH, Stenning SP, *et al*. Perioperative chemotherapy versus surgery alone for resectable gastroesophageal cancer. *N. Engl. J. Med.* 2006; 355: 11–20.

FURTHER READING

Allum WH, Griffin SM, Watson A and Colin-Jones D (on behalf of the Association of Upper Gastrointestinal Surgeons of Great Britain and Ireland, the British Society of Gastroenterology, and the British Association of Surgical Oncology). Guidelines for the management of oesophageal and gastric cancer. *Gut* 2002; 50 (Suppl. 5): v1–v23. Full text available at http://www.bsg.org.uk/

2.2.3 Rare gastric tumours

Leiomyoma

This is a benign tumour of smooth muscle. Most tumours less than 2 cm are asymptomatic. In contrast, tumours greater than 2 cm may ulcerate and cause profuse gastrointestinal haemorrhage. Submucosal endoscopic biopsy is often non-diagnostic, but leiomyomas have a characteristic endoscopic appearance with central ulceration. Around 1% are malignant. Endoscopic ultrasound can also be used to further characterise the lesion. If bleeding occurs, surgical resection is indicated.

Gastric and MALT lymphomas

Around 3–6% of gastric tumours are lymphomas, predominantly extranodal B-cell non-Hodgkin type. Low-grade lymphomas are associated with *Helicobacter pylori* infection in 72–98% of cases, *H. pylori* infection probably having resulted in the migration of B cells into the gastric mucosa as the stomach is usually devoid of mucosal-associated lymphoid tissue (MALT).

Most patients present over the age of 50 years, with non-specific dyspepsia, nausea and vomiting. There are usually no physical signs and weight loss is rare. There may be no macroscopic abnormality or simply gastritis. Endoscopic biopsies are needed to make the diagnosis.

Long-term follow-up studies show that eradication of *H. pylori* can cause resolution of most low-grade MALT lymphomas confined to the mucosa. Non-responsive MALT lymphomas may have undergone high-grade transformation and require chemotherapy with chlorambucil. Surgery is only necessary for those with complications such as haemorrhage or perforation.

Gastrinoma

Gastrinoma causes multiple duodenal ulcers and is associated with steatorrhoea due to acidic destruction of pancreatic lipase. It may be sporadic or associated with multiple endocrine neoplasia type 1. Sporadic tumours are usually single and found in the duodenal wall or pancreas; 50% are benign. Treatment is by resection or with high-dose proton pump inhibitor. There is a good 10-year prognosis.

FURTHER READING

Banks PM. Gastrointestinal lymphoproliferative disorders. *Histopathology* 2007; 50: 42–54.

Hong SS, Jung HY, Choi KD, *et al.* A prospective analysis of low-grade gastric malt lymphoma after *Helicobacter pylori* eradication. *Helicobacter* 2006; 11: 569–73.

2.2.4 Rare causes of gastrointestinal haemorrhage

Dieulafoy lesion

This is due to an artery in the submucosa with an overlying mucosal defect that results in massive upper gastrointestinal haemorrhage. It is usually found within 6 cm of the gastro-oesophageal junction. The mean age at presentation is 50 years. The lesion may be missed at endoscopy when air inflates the stomach. Endoscopic banding can be employed to stop the bleeding, but some require surgical oversewing of the artery.

Vascular ectasia (angiodysplasia)

These are dilated, distorted, thin-walled vessels which are usually multiple (Fig. 32). They occur anywhere along the gastrointestinal tract, but commonly in the caecum and descending colon. They usually present in middle age, most typically with iron-deficiency anaemia, but 15% are associated with massive bleeding. Treatments include medical therapies such as oestrogens, endoscopic electrocoagulation and surgical resection (Fig. 33). They are associated with aortic stenosis (for reasons unknown).

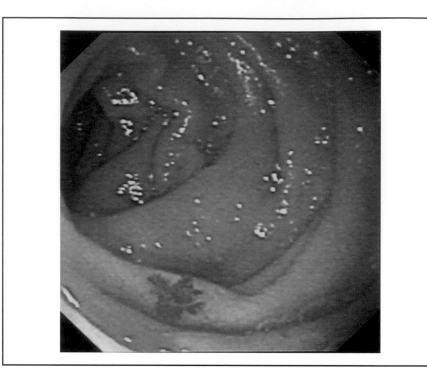

▲ **Fig. 32** Angiodysplastic lesion found in the duodenum of a patient with severe iron-deficiency anaemia.

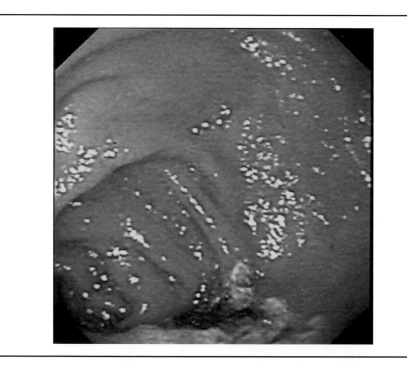

▲ **Fig. 33** Appearance of angiodysplastic lesion following argon plasma coagulation therapy.

Hereditary haemorrhagic telangiectasia

This is an autosomal dominant condition associated with skin and mucosal haemorrhage. The vascular lesions commonly occur in the stomach and small bowel and lead to recurrent gastrointestinal haemorrhage and transfusion-dependent anaemia. Cutaneous manifestations include telangiectasia over the lips, fingers and oral mucosa. Treatment is with oestrogens.

Meckel's diverticulum

This congenital abnormality is present in 0.3–3% of the population. It is found on the antimesenteric border of the small bowel within 100 cm of the ileocaecal valve. Most are asymptomatic, but 80% contain ectopic gastric mucosa. Complications include haemorrhage (melaena or dark red blood per rectum), obstruction or intussusception. The diagnosis is made by small bowel enema or technetium-99 scan (which detects parietal cells).

2.3 Small bowel disease

2.3.1 Malabsorption

Malabsorption occurs when the constituents of the small intestine are either transported too quickly or not adequately broken down, or there is reduced capacity for absorption. The most common cause of malabsorption in the UK is coeliac disease (see Section 2.3.2); other causes are described below.

2.3.1.1 Bacterial overgrowth

Aetiology/pathophysiology/pathology

Akin to fresh water in a free-flowing river compared with stagnant water in a pond, bacterial overgrowth is promoted by any condition that impedes the normal flow of intestinal contents. The normal small intestine is not sterile but houses $<10^4$ organisms/mL; in bacterial overgrowth this rises to 10^4–10^9 organisms/mL. The mechanisms by which such bacterial overgrowth produces diarrhoea (usually steatorrhoea) are not completely clear, but deconjugation of bile salts by bacteria may interfere with fat

micelle formation and thus impair fat absorption. Other mechanisms may include direct damage to the enterocytes/mucosal surface or brush border enzymes, or indirect damage by deconjugated bile salts. Bacteria also metabolise vitamin B_{12}.

Epidemiology

Incidence and prevalence are unknown but may be decreasing as a result of reduced surgical intervention for peptic ulcer disease.

Clinical presentation

Common

Chronic diarrhoea or steatorrhoea.

Uncommon

Neurological disorder, eg peripheral neuropathy, subacute combined degeneration of the spinal cord (secondary to B_{12} deficiency). Folic acid deficiency in the elderly is sometimes the only indicator of malabsorption.

Physical signs

None due to bacterial overgrowth *per se*. Look for neuropathy and associated diseases, eg Crohn's, previous peptic ulcer disease surgery.

Investigation

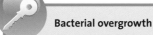

Bacterial overgrowth

Be alert to the diagnosis in patients developing diarrhoea who have a predisposition for this problem, eg those with structural abnormalities of the small bowel.

Glucose or lactulose hydrogen breath test

This is the usual diagnostic test. Glucose is absorbed completely in the upper small bowel; if bacteria are present they will metabolise glucose to hydrogen and methane

and cause a rise in breath hydrogen or methane. Lactulose is a non-absorbable synthetic disaccharide that is metabolised by colonic bacteria. Bacterial overgrowth of the small bowel causes an early rise, but false positives may occur with rapid small intestinal transit.

Jejunal aspiration and culture

The gold standard for diagnosis, but invasive and rarely used, although it does give bacterial sensitivities that can be useful for optimising antibiotic regimens in those patients with resistant bacteria.

Small bowel follow-through

Small bowel radiology is indicated to look for diverticula in those patients who do not have a known underlying structural small bowel abnormality.

Differential diagnosis

Other causes of diarrhoea and steatorrhoea (see Sestions 1.1.3 and 1.4.2).

Treatment

Antibiotic treatment with the aim of suppressing 'bad' bacteria in favour of 'good' bacteria. Augmentin (co-amoxiclav) or a 5-fluoroquinolone has been shown to be effective. Some patients require cyclical rotating courses of antibiotics. Vitamin B_{12} injections may be required.

Complications

Malnutrition, neuropathy and deficiencies of fat-soluble vitamins.

Prognosis

Most of the predisposing conditions are not correctable, so is often a chronic recurring condition unless cyclical antibiotics are employed. Morbidity probably mostly due to lack of diagnosis. Unlikely to have any effect on mortality.

Disease associations

See Table 30.

TABLE 30 CAUSES OF BACTERIAL OVERGROWTH		
Anatomical	**Functional**	**Immune deficiency**
Surgical blind loops	Autonomic neuropathy	Hypogammaglobulinaemia
Billroth II	Amyloid	Achlorhydria
Roux-en-Y	Diabetes mellitus	
Jejunal diverticula	Systemic sclerosis	
Strictures		
Crohn's disease		
Radiation enteritis		
Enterocolic fistulae		

FURTHER READING

Quigley EM and Quera R. Small intestinal bacterial overgrowth: roles of antibiotics, prebiotics, and probiotics. *Gastroenterology* 2006; 130 (2 Suppl. 1): S78–S90.

Singh VV and Toskes PP. Small bowel bacterial overgrowth: presentation, diagnosis, and treatment. *Curr. Treat. Options Gastroenterol.* 2004; 7: 19–28.

2.3.1.2 Other causes of malabsorption

Chronic pancreatitis/pancreatic insufficiency

May occur following repeated acute attacks of pancreatitis, alcohol being the most common culprit, or without any identifiable cause. Steatorrhoea develops when less than 10% of pancreatic exocrine function remains. Diagnosis is made by a combination of imaging and dynamic function tests. Treatment is with pancreatic enzyme supplements titrated against response.

Whipple's disease

A rare disease caused by *Tropheryma whippelii* that usually occurs in white middle-aged or elderly men. It is characterised by malabsorption, migratory polyarthritis, anaemia and weight loss. Neurological and cardiac involvement may occur, as well as pigmentation and clubbing. Jejunal biopsy shows large 'foamy' macrophages in the lamina propria which contain material positive for periodic acid–Schiff (PAS) stain. Treatment is with sulfamethoxazole and trimethoprim for 1 year. Prognosis is good.

Tropical sprue

Occurs in residents of the tropics (India, Asia, Central America) but is rare in Africa. It usually follows an acute diarrhoeal illness. There is persistent bacterial overgrowth in the small bowel, resulting typically in steatorrhoea, weight loss, anaemia, hypoproteinaemia and glossitis. Small bowel biopsy (jejunal) shows partial villous atrophy and round cell infiltration of the lamina propria. The mortality is 10–20% within months if untreated, but it responds readily to tetracycline 250 mg qds and folic acid 5 mg tds.

Giardiasis

Caused by the flagellated protozoan *Giardia lamblia*. It is usually contracted abroad, although it can occur in UK. It has faecal–oral transmission and is characterised by persistent diarrhoea after an acute diarrhoeal episode. Malabsorption is unusual but can occur. Diagnosis is made by finding trophozoites in jejunal aspiration and biopsy (stool culture is less sensitive). Tinidazole 2 g as a single dose or metronidazole 800 mg tds for 3 days is very effective.

Hypolactasia

Primary hypolactasia is common in most races apart from northern Europeans. Lactase, a brush border enzyme that breaks lactose into glucose and galactose, disappears after weaning. Subsequent lactose ingestion (milk) causes an osmotic diarrhoea. It is diagnosed on clinical grounds or by lactose hydrogen breath test.

Secondary hypolactasia can be caused by anything that damages the small bowel mucosa (eg viral gastroenteritis, coeliac disease, Crohn's disease) and reverses on treatment of the underlying disorder.

Short bowel syndrome

Malabsorption occurs when the length of effective small intestine is reduced to less than 100 cm by surgical resection, mesenteric infarction, severe Crohn's disease or radiation injury. Absorptive capacity is overwhelmed and diarrhoea and malabsorption ensue. Adaptation occurs, with improvement for up to 2 years. The colon contributes to energy supplies via fermentation of non-absorbed dietary fibre to short-chain fatty acids which are then absorbed. Treatment is difficult and includes dietary modification, attempts to slow intestinal transport and increase absorption, parenteral nutrition, and bowel transplantation in severe cases.

Post gastric surgery

Frank malabsorption following gastric surgery is rare. Iron deficiency is common. The cause is multifactoral and includes hypoacidity, chronic bleeding from friable anastomosis, and decreased intake. Vitamin B_{12} deficiency may also occur due to lack of intrinsic factor or bacterial overgrowth. Fat malabsorption is caused by an impaired pancreatic response due to bypassing of the duodenum in a Billroth II gastrectomy, vagal denervation, or rapid gastric emptying preventing optimal mixing with pancreatic juices.

FURTHER READING

Nightingale J and Woodward JM (on behalf of the Small Bowel and Nutrition Committee of the British Society of Gastroenterology). Guidelines for management of patients with a short bowel. *Gut* 2006; 55 (Suppl. 4): iv1–iv12. Full text available at http://www.bsg.org.uk/

2.3.2 Coeliac disease

Aetiology/pathophysiology/ pathology

Coeliac disease or gluten-sensitive enteropathy is a state of heightened immunological responsiveness to ingested gluten in genetically susceptible individuals. It is characterised by damage of the small intestinal mucosa due to intolerance to a group of proteins present in wheat, barley and rye. The aetiology is unknown but probably requires both environmental and genetic factors: 10–12% of first-degree relatives of an affected individual have the disease; 85–90% of patients carry major histocompatibility complex (MHC) class II markers HLA-DR3 and HLA-DQ2, and the remainder are DQ8 positive (these HLA markers are present in a large proportion of the population and less than 0.1% of individuals with this haplotype actually develop coeliac disease, but it is not possible to have coeliac disease without one of these HLA markers). Tissue transglutaminase has recently been identified as the autoantigen towards which endomysial antibodies are directed.

Gliadin peptides are rich in glutamic acid residues that are modified by tissue transglutaminase and

presented to intraepithelial T cells by antigen-presenting cells via the HLA-DQ2 molecule. Activation of T cells results in patchy damage to the small intestinal mucosa, with the proximal small bowel more severely affected. Changes in the intestinal lining are graded using the modified Marsh criteria shown in Table 31.

Epidemiology

Coeliac disease was once thought to be rare but has been shown by large screening studies in Europe and the USA to affect 1 in 100–200 people. It is rare in Africa and has not been described in China or the Caribbean. It occurs more commonly in females (2:1). In adults, diagnosis peaks in the fourth and fifth decades in women, and the fifth and sixth decades in men.

> Coeliac disease may present for the first time in the seventh or eighth decade of life.

Clinical presentation

Symptoms and signs are as shown in Table 32.

TABLE 31 MODIFIED MARSH CRITERIA FOR HISTOLOGICAL CLASSFICATION OF COELIAC DISEASE

Marsh grade	Histological findings
0	Normal
1	Increased intraepithelial lymphocytes
2	1+ crypt hyperplasia
3a	2+ partial villous atrophy
3b	2+ subtotal villous atrophy
3c	2+ total villous atrophy

TABLE 32 SYMPTOMS AND SIGNS OF COELIAC DISEASE

Common	Less common	Rare
Anaemia[1,2]: iron, folate or mixed deficiency, often found by chance Diarrhoea[1,2]: typically pale, bulky, offensive and difficult to flush Weight loss[1,2]/failure to thrive[1]/short stature Irritable bowel-type symptoms[2] (eg distension, pain, bloating, borborygmi) Anorexia, nausea, vomiting[1] Aphthous oral ulceration, glossitis, stomatitis General malaise, lethargy Mood change[1,2], anxiety, depression	Infertility/amenorrhoea Bone pain: osteomalacia, osteoporosis Dermatitis herpetiformis	Neurological: peripheral neuropathy, cerebellar ataxia, etc. Tetany: hypocalcaemia Rickets Bruising and night-blindness: deficiencies of fat-soluble vitamins A and K Constipation

1. Commonest signs and symptoms in infancy.
2. Commonest signs and symptoms in adults.

> The diagnosis of coeliac disease should be seriously considered in any patient with diarrhoea/steatorrhoea or with iron- or folate-deficiency anaemia.

Investigation

The most important issue is to have a high index of suspicion for the diagnosis.

Blood tests

An FBC may show anaemia (iron and/or folate deficiency) and the blood film a dimorphic population of red blood cells with Howell–Jolly bodies (associated hyposplenism). Occasionally there is isolated B_{12} or folic acid deficiency. Some newly diagnosed patients have raised transaminases, but these usually normalise after treatment.

Serology

Anti-gliadin antibodies are commonly present but have a lower sensitivity than other serological markers. The combination of anti-endomysial antibody (anti-EMA) and anti-tissue transglutaminase antibody (anti-tTG) has a sensitivity and specificity above 95%. Some patients have an associated IgA deficiency that can render these tests negative as they are IgA based. However, one of the anti-gliadin antibodies is IgG based and there are IgG versions of anti-EMA and anti-tTG.

Histology

Histological examination of small bowel biopsies remains the gold standard for diagnosing coeliac disease, and should be performed if the condition is suspected whilst the subject is on a gluten-containing diet. Previously jejunal material was obtained via a Crosby capsule, but now the standard technique is to obtain four duodenal biopsies because of the patchy nature of the intestinal findings.

Barium follow-through

This is often abnormal but is not usually needed to make the diagnosis. The normal fine feathery appearance of the mucosa is replaced by a coarser pattern (transverse barring) or a tubular featureless appearance in severe disease.

Differential diagnosis

- If diarrhoea: giardiasis, infection, inflammatory bowel disease.

- If abdominal pain and/or weight loss: Crohn's disease and thyrotoxicosis.

- If steatorrhoea: exocrine pancreatic insufficiency.

- If iron-deficiency anaemia: consider other reasons for blood loss.

Other causes of villous atrophy include giardiasis, hypogammaglobulinaemia, bacterial overgrowth, tropical sprue, cows' milk sensitivity, Whipple's disease, lymphoma and NSAIDs.

Treatment

Gluten-free diet

Strict withdrawal of gluten from the diet is advocated: 85% of cases respond to this and relapse on its reintroduction. Physicians and dietitians should be involved in educating the patient about the condition, and membership of Coeliac UK encouraged. Compliance can be assessed using serial antibody measurements, which usually diminish once gluten is withdrawn from the diet. The small intestinal mucosa may take many years to normalise, if at all, and therefore routine follow-up duodenal biopsies may not be useful.

> Persistence of anti-EMA 6 weeks after starting dietary therapy suggests non-compliance.

Dietary supplementation

Iron, folate, vitamin D and calcium supplementation may be required at diagnosis depending on the degree of abnormality and symptoms.

Non-responsive coeliac disease

Some patients do not respond adequately to a gluten-free diet and this may indicate the presence of associated conditions or complications. The most common reason for continued symptoms in coeliac disease is continued gluten exposure and therefore reassessment of the diet (perhaps best performed by a dietitian) is essential. Associated conditions include exocrine pancreatic insufficiency (up to one-third), new thyroid disease (1–2%) and lactose intolerance. Alternatively one of the complications may have arisen.

Immunosuppression

In those patients who do not respond to dietary treatment, steroids and other immunosuppressants, such as azathioprine, may be required to induce remission.

> **Important information for patients**
>
> Symptoms of coeliac disease are usually relieved and complications reduced by permanent adoption of strict gluten-free diet: join Coeliac UK (see http://www.coeliac.co.uk/ for details).

TABLE 33 CONDITIONS ASSOCIATED WITH COELIAC DISEASE

Condition	Prevalence of coeliac disease (%)
Dermatitis herpetiformis	70
Type 1 diabetes mellitus	3–7
Thyroid disease	Up to 7
Irritable bowel syndrome	5
Idiopathic dilated cardiomyopathy	3–6
Primary biliary cirrhosis	3
Rheumatoid arthritis	3
Sjögren's syndrome	3
Infertility	2–3
Osteoporosis	3
IgA deficiency	2.5
Epilepsy (with cerebral calcifications)	2.3
Down's syndrome	2

Complications

- Bone disease in up to 40% (osteoporosis and osteomalacia).

- Increased risk of gastrointestinal malignancy (enteropathy-associated T-cell lymphoma, squamous cell carcinoma of the pharynx and oesophagus, and small intestinal adenocarcinoma).

- Hyposplenism: common and related to duration and severity of disease, but rarely causes problems.

- Ulcerative enteritis: a rare complication that may be an early manifestation of malignant lymphoma.

> Osteopenia and osteoporosis are relatively common at diagnosis, but malignant complications are rare.

Prognosis

Mortality

Mortality is increased in coeliac disease, chiefly due to an excess of malignant disease. Adoption of a gluten-free diet appears to protect against this complication and results in a normal lifespan.

Disease associations

Associated diseases are shown in Table 33.

FURTHER READING

Al-Toma A, Verbeek WH and Mulder CJ. Update on the management of refractory coeliac disease. *J. Gastrointest. Liver Dis.* 2007; 16: 57–63.

Ciclitira P. *Guidelines for the Management of Patients with Coeliac Disease*. London: British Society for Gastroenterology, 2002. Full text available at http://www.bsg.org.uk/

Goddard CJ and Gillett HR. Complications of coeliac disease: are all patients at risk? *Postgrad. Med. J.* 2006; 82: 705–12.

2.4 Pancreatic disease

> Diseases of the pancreas provide an enormous challenge to the clinician, and although patients with the more common forms of pancreatic disease (ie acute pancreatitis and pancreatic carcinoma) have historically been managed by surgical teams, there is a growing trend for non-surgical (ie medical) management.

2.4.1 Acute pancreatitis

Aetiology/pathophysiology/pathology

This is an acute inflammatory process of the pancreas with variable involvement of other regional tissues or remote organ systems. Once the process has started, the degree of pancreatic necrosis is variable and in part related to proteolytic autodigestion of the gland.

The most common causes of acute pancreatitis in the UK are gallstones (30–50%) and alcohol (10–40%), but a significant number of cases do not have an immediately obvious cause (15%).

> In the absence of gallstones or alcohol, consider the following rare causes of acute pancreatitis before making an 'idiopathic' diagnosis.
>
> - Drugs: steroids, azathioprine, sulfasalazine, furosemide.
> - Pancreas divisum: congenital malfusion of the dorsal and ventral pancreatic buds.
> - Sphincter of Oddi dysfunction: high pressure sphincter causing duct hypertension.
> - Hypertriglyceridaemia: may be associated with alcohol abuse or diabetes.
> - Hypercalcaemia/hyperparathyroidism.
> - Viral: mumps, coxsackievirus B, Epstein–Barr virus, cytomegalovirus.
> - Hereditary pancreatitis (see Section 2.4.2).
> - Hypothermia: rewarming injury to the pancreas.

Clinical presentation

Common

- Abdominal pain, usually epigastric and radiating through to the back.

- Vomiting.

- Hypovolaemia, circulatory collapse, hypoxia.

Uncommon

Jaundice suggests the presence of an associated cholangitis and raises the probability of gallstones.

Rare

No pain (consider hypothermia).

Physical signs

Common

In mild acute pancreatitis there may be few physical signs. Otherwise expect abdominal/epigastric tenderness or infrequent or absent bowel sounds.

Uncommon

In patients with more severe disease there will be clinical evidence of hypovolaemia and systemic inflammation. Other features may include:

- mental state (the patient may be agitated and delirious);

- tachycardia;

- hypotension;

- fever;

- peripheral cyanosis;

- peritonism.

Rare

Cullen's sign (periumbilical bruising) and Grey Turner's sign (flank bruising) are both associated with severe haemorrhagic pancreatitis.

Investigation/staging

Diagnosis with serum amylase

Serum amylase is diagnostic of pancreatitis if more than three times the upper limit of normal for the laboratory. Alternatives include serum lipase and possibly urinary trypsinogen.

Assessment of severity

Severity can be assessed using the Glasgow/Ranson criteria.

Glasgow/Ranson criteria

Three or more positive criteria, based on initial admission score and subsequent repeat tests over 48 hours, constitutes severe disease.

- Age >55 years.
- White blood cell count >15 × 10⁹/L.
- Glucose >10 mmol/L.
- Urea >16 mmol/L.
- Pao_2 <8 kPa (60 mmHg).
- Calcium <2 mmol/L.
- Albumin <32 g/L.
- Lactate dehydrogenase >600 U/L.
- Aspartate/alanine aminotransferase >100 U/L.

The Acute Physiology and Chronic Health Evaluation (APACHE II) scoring system is used in many intensive care units. An APACHE II score of 9 or more is considered to constitute a severe attack of acute pancreatitis.

A peak C-reactive protein level >210 mg/L in the first 4 days of the attack (or >120 mg/L at the end of the first week) indicates severe disease.

Assessment of cause

An abdominal ultrasound should be performed within 24 hours of admission. This will determine whether there are gallstones present and may demonstrate biliary dilatation, suggesting common bile duct obstruction.

Assessment for complications

Depending on the method of presentation, some patients will undergo abdominal CT as their first imaging investigation to exclude other causes of 'acute abdomen'. A CT with contrast should be performed in cases of severe pancreatitis between 3 and 10 days after admission. In addition to identifying secondary complications such as pseudocyst formation (Fig. 34), the extent of pancreatic necrosis carries prognostic value (Table 34).

Differential diagnosis

This includes perforated peptic ulcer, intestinal ischaemia/infarction, ectopic pregnancy, aortic dissection, myocardial infarction (see Section 1.4.4).

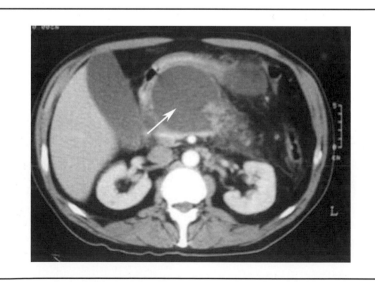

▲ **Fig. 34** Pancreatic pseudocyst complicating acute pancreatitis. The stomach is stretched over the large pseudocyst (arrow). (Courtesy of Dr N.D. Derbyshire, Royal Berkshire Hospital.)

TABLE 34 CONTRAST-ENHANCED CT GRADING OF ACUTE PANCREATITIS

Grade	CT morphology
A	Normal
B	Focal or diffuse gland enlargement; small intrapancreatic fluid collection
C	Any of the above plus peripancreatic inflammatory changes and <30% gland necrosis
D	Any of the above plus single extrapancreatic fluid collection and 30–50% gland necrosis
E	Any of the above plus extensive extrapancreatic fluid collection, pancreatic abscess and >50% gland necrosis

Treatment

Emergency

Resuscitation Intravenous fluids to restore circulating volmue (may require central venous pressure monitoring) and oxygen. Patients with severe pancreatitis (as defined above) should be managed in either a high-dependency unit or an intensive care unit.

Analgesia The pain of acute pancreatitis is usually intense and requires opiate analgesia. Pethidine is usually used because it has less effect on the sphincter of Oddi than morphine.

Nutrition Although historically patients with acute pancreatitis were fasted with gastric aspiration ('drip and suck'), early nasojejunal feeding is now favoured once vomiting has settled.

Antibiotics Use of 'blind' broad-spectrum antibiotics is controversial, although recent studies have suggested a reduction in septic complications. Antibiotics should be used in cases of proven infection or organ failure, with a third-generation cephalosporin generally recommended.

Short-term

Endoscopic retrograde cholangiopancreatography (ERCP) If gallstones are present on ultrasound or if the patient has clinical features of cholangitis (fever, jaundice), early ERCP (ie within the first 24 hours) should be considered on the principle that early relief of biliary obstruction will reduce complications. If this is not performed within 24–48 hours, oedema of the papilla makes ERCP technically difficult. ERCP can also be employed in pseudocyst drainage if there is communication with the pancreatic duct.

Endoscopic ultrasound (EUS) The advent of EUS has enhanced endoscopic interventions for pancreatic disease. A pseudocyst that does not resolve spontaneously within 6 weeks usually needs draining to prevent complications (infection, rupture or bleeding). This can be done into the stomach using EUS guidance, which identifies a suitable tissue plane and helps avoid vessels in the area (Fig. 35).

EUS may also reveal a cause for acute pancreatitis that cannot be identified by other imaging modalities, eg microlithiasis, small tumours or cysts.

Other Surgery may be indicated in cases of infected necrosis. Pancreatic abscess may require CT-guided drainage.

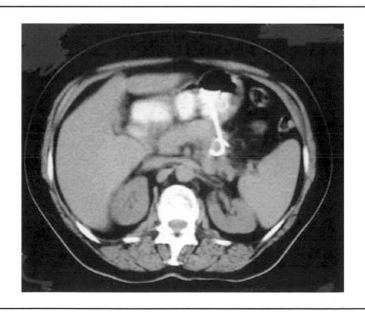

▲ **Fig. 35** Drainage of a pancreatic pseudocyst into the stomach showing the internal transgastric drain *in situ*. (Courtesy of Dr N.D. Derbyshire, Royal Berkshire Hospital.)

Long-term

Management of the appropriate risk factor helps to prevent recurrent attacks:

- abstinence from alcohol;

- early cholecystectomy if gallstones are confirmed to be the underlying cause;

- control lipids/calcium.

Complications

Common

- Pancreatic pseudocyst/abscess (5%): persistent pain and/or fever suggests the development of a pancreatic pseudocyst or abscess, as does a persistently raised amylase.

- Paralytic ileus.

- Hypovolaemic shock.

- Renal failure.

- Hypocalcaemia.

- Hypoxia.

Uncommon

- Portal vein/mesenteric thrombosis.

- Adult respiratory distress syndrome.

- Ascites.

Ascites due to pancreatitis has a high amylase content.

Rare

External pancreatic fistulae may follow percutaneous drainage of pseudocyst.

Prognosis

Thirty per cent of patients have recurrent attacks, which are more likely in pancreatitis related to alcohol consumption. Overall

TABLE 35 PROGNOSIS FROM ACUTE PANCREATITIS

Scoring system	Mortality (%)
Glasgow/Ranson criteria[1]	
<2	5
3–5	10
>6	60
APACHE II[2]	
<9	'low'
>13	'high'

1. Scored at 48 hours from the onset of symptoms: sensitivity 57–85%; specificity 68–85%.
2. Can be scored at any time: sensitivity at admission 34–70%, at 48 hours <50%; specificity at admission 76–98%, at 48 hours 100%.

prognosis may be worse in idiopathic pancreatitis.

Morbidity and mortality

This depends on the severity of the attack (Table 35).

Prevention

Primary

Other than a reduction in alcohol consumption there is little scope for primary prevention of acute pancreatitis.

Secondary

- Cholecystectomy.

- Abstinence from alcohol.

- Management of risk factors.

FURTHER READING

Whitcomb DC. Clinical practice: acute pancreatitis. *N. Engl. J. Med.* 2006; 354: 2142–50.

- - - - - - - - - - - - - - - - - - - -

Working Party of the British Society of Gastroenterology, Association of Surgeons of Great Britain and Ireland, Pancreatic Society of Great Britain and Ireland and Association of Upper GI Surgeons of Great Britain and Ireland. UK guidelines for the management of acute pancreatitis. *Gut* 2005; 54 (Suppl. 3): iii1–iii9. Full text available at http://www.bsg.org.uk/

2.4.2 Chronic pancreatitis

Aetiology/pathophysiology/pathology

Chronic pancreatitis is defined as a progressive inflammatory condition of the pancreas characterised by irreversible changes that typically cause pain and/or permanent loss of both endocrine and exocrine function. This evolution usually occurs over a period of several years. Clinically, this helps to distinguish between acute first-onset pancreatitis, recurrent acute pancreatitis and chronic pancreatitis. However, it is often difficult to classify pancreatitis: histology is not routinely used, but it does remain the gold standard for the early stage of chronic pancreatitis, where there is loss of normal acinar cells, fibrosis and lymphocytic infiltrate.

Cause of chronic pancreatitis (TIGAR O)

- Toxic/metabolic: most notably alcohol (>60% of cases) and hyperlipidaemia.
- Idiopathic: accounts for 10–30% of cases.
- Genetic: cystic fibrosis gene mutations, cationic trypsinogen gene mutations (*PRSS1*) and serine

- protease inhibitor Kazal type 1 (*SPINK1*) mutations.
- Autoimmune: more common in Far East.
- Recurrent and severe acute pancreatitis: progressive parenchymal tissue damage.
- Obstruction: congenital malformations, eg annular pancreas.

duct or development of pancreatic carcinoma.

> Both exocrine and endocrine insufficiency may be absent in mild chronic pancreatitis: their presence indicates substantial pancreatic damage.

Epidemiology

Rare. Estimated incidence varies between 1.6 and 23 per 100,000, with prevalence about four times higher.

Clinical presentation

Common

Abdominal pain, typically epigastric radiating through to the back. It is often precipitated by eating fatty foods or drinking alcohol.

Uncommon

- Exocrine pancreatic insufficiency: steatorrhoea and weight loss.

- Endocrine pancreatic insufficiency: diabetes.

Rare

Jaundice: due to either fibrosis encroaching on the common bile

Physical signs

Common

There are no specific physical signs until there has been sufficient destruction of the gland to cause pancreatic failure (either exocrine or endocrine).

Uncommon

Erythema ab igne may be evident on the anterior abdominal wall in patients with chronic pancreatic pain.

Investigation/staging

Serum amylase is often normal or at most only modestly elevated and therefore only of value during attacks of acute abdominal pain to exclude acute-on-chronic pancreatitis (although serum amylase level may not reach diagnostic levels).

Tests of pancreatic anatomy

Abdominal radiograph, ultrasound and CT Plain abdominal radiograph may show pancreatic calcification. Ultrasound has a sensitivity of about 70% for detecting parenchymal pancreatic changes via transabdominal scanning, but the pancreas is often obscured by overlying bowel gas. On abdominal CT, the features of chronic pancreatitis include parenchymal calcification, duct irregularities and cysts.

Endoscopic retrograde cholangiopancreatography (ERCP)/magnetic resonance cholangiopancreatography (MRCP) Chronic pancreatitis can be classified using the Cambridge system, which looks at main pancreatic duct integrity, duct size dilatation, presence of calculi or stones and any cavities. It can be applied to ultrasound, CT, ERCP and MRCP, with the latter having the advantage of being non-invasive, although early changes may be missed because the duct is not filled by contrast injection. ERCP (Fig. 36) has the option of therapeutic intervention.

Endoscopic ultrasound (EUS) This is less invasive than ERCP and therefore has fewer complications

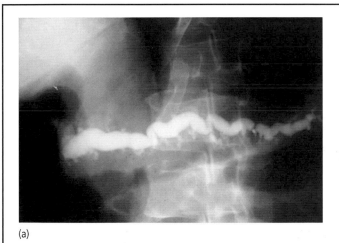

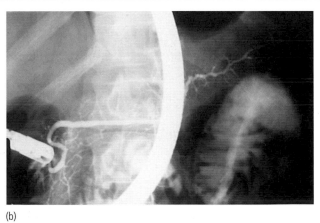

(a)

(b)

▲ **Fig. 36** Chronic pancreatitis shown on ERCP: (**a**) dilated pancreatic duct with loss of side branches in severe disease compared with (**b**) minimal duct changes.

whilst allowing high-resolution images of the pancreatic parenchyma and the ductal system. EUS also has therapeutic capabilities (see below under analgesia).

Tests of exocrine pancreatic function

Deterioration in exocrine function occurs when >90% of pancreatic tissue or >85% of lipase output is lost. There are many methods of assessing exocrine pancreatic function, which can be divided into direct and indirect tests (see Section 3.2 for further information).

Tests of endocrine pancreatic function

Glucose tolerance test, but note that this is not helpful in staging chronic pancreatitis.

Differential diagnosis

- Of pain: peptic ulcer, pancreatic cancer.

- Of steatorrhoea and weight loss: coeliac disease, small bowel bacterial overgrowth, giardiasis.

Treatment

Pancreatic enzyme replacement

Preparations such as Creon and Pancrex often improve both the pain and the malabsorption associated with chronic pancreatitis. Some patients have a partial response and may require addition of acid suppression to reduce enzyme destruction by the stomach.

Analgesia

Where pain is the dominant feature, opiate analgesia and local approaches such as coeliac axis block may be necessary. EUS can be employed to guide coeliac plexus blockade.

Others

Pancreatic diabetes has the same complication rate as any other type of diabetes and therefore requires global assessment: although hyperglycaemia may be relatively mild, early treatment with insulin is often useful. Ensure abstinence from alcohol.

Antioxidants

There is some evidence that antioxidant therapy can improve pain and morbidity associated with chronic pancreatitis (particularly alcohol related).

Complications

Common

Malabsorption and diabetes.

Uncommon

Common bile duct obstruction.

Rare

Pancreatic carcinoma.

Prognosis

Morbidity

Although diabetes and malabsorption can be treated, chronic pain is a major source of morbidity with associated loss of employment, depression and opiate dependence.

Mortality

Survival is reduced in all causes of chronic pancreatitis. Outcomes are often worse in alcoholic chronic pancreatitis, with death in this group being due to many different causes.

Prevention

Secondary

Abstinence from alcohol along with medical management as outlined above will usually lead to clinical stabilisation.

FURTHER READING

Ahmed SA, Wray C, Rilo HL, *et al.* Chronic pancreatitis: recent advances and ongoing challenges. *Curr. Probl. Surg.* 2006; 43: 127–238.

- - - - - - - - - - - - - - - - - -

Gupta V and Toskes PP. Diagnosis and management of chronic pancreatitis. *Postgrad. Med. J.* 2005; 81: 491–7.

2.4.3 Pancreatic cancer

Aetiology/pathophysiology/pathology

Most primary malignant tumours of the pancreas are adenocarcinoma. Risk factors include increasing age, male sex, smoking, alcohol, chronic pancreatitis, diabetes (within 2 years of diagnosis of type 2 diabetes mellitus) and hereditary pancreatitis.

Epidemiology

Pancreatic carcinoma is the fourth commonest gastointestinal tumour. Its incidence is increasing in the Western world, in the range of 5–10 per 100,000. Male to female ratio is 1.3:1. It is rare in patients under 45 years old.

Clinical presentation

Common

- Painless cholestatic jaundice associated with varying degrees of pruritus, pale stools and dark urine due to common bile duct obstruction.

- Weight loss.

- Abdominal pain.

Uncommon

- Vomiting (from duodenal obstruction).

- Malignant ascites.

- Unexplained exocrine pancreatic insufficiency.

- Unexplained episode of acute pancreatitis.

Rare

- Venous thrombosis (thrombophlebitis migrans).

- Diabetes.

Physical signs

Common

Jaundice and cachexia.

Uncommon

- Palpable gallbladder (Courvoisier's sign).

- Palpable mass.

- Ascites.

Investigation/staging

Blood tests

Routine blood tests show non-specific changes related to biliary obstruction. The pancreaticobiliary tumour marker CA19-9 may be elevated but is not specific to pancreatic tumours.

Non-invasive imaging

Abdominal ultrasound May show a dilated biliary tree. A pancreatic mass may be demonstrated, but the absence of a mass on ultrasound does not exclude a pancreatic malignancy. Dilatation of both the common bile duct and the pancreatic duct is highly suggestive of a carcinoma of the pancreatic head ('double duct' sign).

> The absence of gallstones on ultrasound in a patient presenting with acute cholestasis and a dilated biliary tree suggests the presence of a common bile duct stricture due to a carcinoma of the pancreas or cholangiocarcinoma.

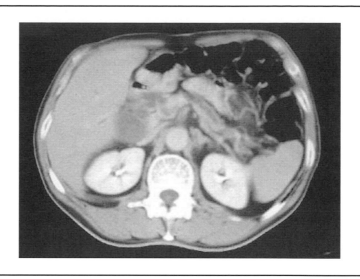

▲ **Fig. 37** CT scan showing carcinoma of the head of the pancreas with distal pancreatic duct dilatation. (Courtesy of Dr N.D. Derbyshire, Royal Berkshire Hospital.)

Abdominal CT or MRI CT scanning is useful for demonstrating the mass and for staging, ie demonstration of invasion into important local structures or evidence of distant metastases (Fig. 37).

Invasive imaging

Endoscopic retrograde cholangiopancreatography (ERCP) Duodenoscopy allows assessment of the ampulla of Vater and identification and biopsy of a lesion if present. ERCP allows diagnosis and placement of an endobiliary stent to allow relief from biliary obstruction in patients (the majority) who are unsuitable for surgical resection. Carries a significant morbidity and mortality.

Percutaneous transhepatic cholangiography (PTC) For cases where ERCP has failed or is not possible, eg previous surgery such as Polya gastrectomy or Roux-en-Y biliary reconstruction; also allows placement of an endobiliary stent.

Endoscopic ultrasound (EUS) CT and transabdominal ultrasound can miss lesions <2 cm in size. EUS is particularly good at detecting these

and has the capability of directing tissue sampling by either fine-needle aspiration or biopsy. The fact that it has higher resolution than other imaging modalities allows clearer definition of local invasion into vascular structures and therefore resectability.

CT-guided biopsy Useful in selected cases where the diagnosis remains obscure and where surgical resection might be considered if a positive diagnosis of adenocarcinoma is confirmed, but there is a risk of seeding along the track.

> Pancreatic tumours are very fibrotic and biopsy has a higher sensitivity than aspiration cytology.

Differential diagnosis

- Of acute cholestasis: choledocholithiasis, intrahepatic cholestasis (eg drug reaction).

- Of pancreatic mass: ampullary carcinoma (tumour arising from the ampulla of Vater), which has a better prognosis.

Treatment

This depends on suitability for surgery. Patients who have resectable disease and who will be operated on in a timely fashion may not require stenting. Routine preoperative biliary decompression has not been shown to be beneficial.

Short-term

Those with extremely symptomatic jaundice may require stenting prior to surgery, but the route of delivery and type of stent is controversial. The British Society of Gastroenterology guidelines suggest plastic stenting via ERCP, although many centres prefer metal stenting via PTC as there is a lower risk of pancreatitis and therefore less risk of unnecessary delay.

Long-term or according to stage

Curative surgery In about 20% of patients, pancreaticoduodenectomy (Whipple's procedure) offers the possibility of a surgical cure. No other form of therapy is associated with long-term survival.

Palliative surgery Surgery may still be beneficial in patients with advanced disease by providing combined biliary and gastroduodenal bypass. Can be performed laparoscopically in some cases in some centres.

Chemotherapy/radiotherapy Oncological therapies in pancreatic carcinoma are used to help control symptoms and improve quality of life. Multimodal therapy (external beam irradiation combined with 5-flurouracil chemotherapy) has been shown to have no advantage over chemotherapy alone, providing minimal survival advantage (in the range of weeks). In recent studies gemcitabine (a pyrimidine nucleoside analogue) has been shown to improve quality of life, and there appears to be a modest

but significant increase in response rate and survival using regimens containing this agent.

Palliative measures Relief of jaundice and pain control are the main objectives in patients with advanced disease and many require opiate analgesia. Anorexia and weight loss remain major problems.

Nutritional issues The addition of pancreatic enzyme supplements (such as Creon) has been shown to improve quality of life and reduce cachexia in patients with advanced pancreatic cancer.

Prognosis

Morbidity

Most patients with pancreatic cancer have incurable disease at presentation and will experience pain in addition to progressive anorexia and weight loss.

Mortality

Of individuals presenting with carcinoma of the pancreas, 90% are dead within 1 year.

FURTHER READING

Choti MA. Adjuvant therapy for pancreatic cancer: the debate continues. *N. Engl. J. Med.* 2004; 350: 1249–51.

- - - - - - - - - - - - - - - - - - -

Pancreatic Section of the British Society of Gastroenterology, Pancreatic Society of Great Britain and Ireland, Association of Upper Gastrointestinal Surgeons of Great Britain and Ireland, Royal College of Pathologists and Special Interest Group for Gastro-Intestinal Radiology. Guidelines for the management of patients with pancreatic cancer, periampullary and ampullary carcinomas. *Gut* 2005; 54 (Suppl. 5): v1–v16. Full text available at http://www.bsg.org.uk/

2.4.4 Neuroendocrine tumours

Aetiology/pathophysiology/ pathology

Tumours arising from the specialised neuroendocrine tissue of the pancreas or intestine. They are rare but important differentials for a variety of clinical syndromes including pancreatic mass lesions.

Epidemiology and genetic background

All neuroendocrine tumours are rare. They may occur as part of several familial cancer syndromes, notably multiple endocrine neoplasia (MEN) type 1, MEN type 2, neurofibromatosis type 1 and von Hippel–Lindau syndrome.

Clinical presentation and physical signs

These vary depending on tumour type (Table 36).

Investigation/staging

Stool weight

This is performed on a normal diet and then repeated fasting to distinguish secretory from osmotic diarrhoea.

The diarrhoea associated with hormone excess is characteristically secretory rather than osmotic (ie not diminished by fasting).

Blood tests

Serum chromogranin A has an uncertain role but is produced by all cells derived from the neural crest and may be raised in any neuroendocrine tumour. Most neuroendocrine hormones can now be identified on a fasting serum sample. In the case of gastrin it is

TABLE 36 NEUROENDOCRINE TUMOUR TYPE AND COMMON SYMPTOM COMPLEX

Tumour type	Symptoms
Insulinoma	Confusion, sweating, dizziness, weakness
Gastrinoma (Zollinger–Ellison syndrome)	Severe peptic ulceration and diarrhoea
Glucagonoma	Necrolytic migratory erythema, diabetes, weight loss, stomatitis, flushing
VIPoma (Wermer–Morrison syndrome)	Profuse diarrhoea and hypokalaemia
Somatostatinoma	Cholelithiasis, weight loss, diarrhoea, diabetes
Non-functioning	Pancreatic mass

VIP, vasoactive intestinal polypeptide.

important that the patient is not taking acid-suppressing medication at the time of testing.

Pancreatic imaging

In most instances the clinical presentation of neuroendocrine tumours of the pancreas will be due to the systemic effect of the secreted hormone. Identification of the tumour is important as, with the exception of insulinomas, a significant proportion of these lesions are malignant. Spiral CT, MRI and increasingly endoscopic and intraoperative ultrasound are used.

Octreotide scan

Radiolabelled somatostatin binds to receptors on many neuroendocrine tumour cells and can help to localise primary and secondary tumour deposits.

Treatment

Long-term or according to stage

Surgical resection is probably the best treatment if a focal tumour can be identified and the patient is fit enough. Medical treatment depends on the secreted hormone.

- Gastrinoma: high-dose proton pump inhibitors improve both the pain and the diarrhoea.

- Insulinoma: dietary advice, diazoxide, octreotide.

- VIPoma: octreotide.

- Glucagonoma: octreotide.

Prognosis

With the exception of insulinoma, two-thirds of the other tumour types will be histologically malignant. However, with improved medical therapy (proton pump inhibitors and octreotide) these may still follow a relatively indolent course.

FURTHER READING

Kulke MH. New developments in the treatment of gastrointestinal neuroendocrine tumours. *Curr. Oncol. Rep.* 2007; 9: 177–83.

- - - - - - - - - - - - - - - -

Ramage JK, Davies AHG, Ardill J, *et al.* (on behalf of UKNETwork for neuroendocrine tumours). Guidelines for the management of gastroenteropancreatic neuroendocrine (including carcinoid) tumours. *Gut* 2005; 54 (Suppl. 4): iv1–iv16. Full text available at http://www.bsg.org.uk/

2.5 Biliary disease

2.5.1 Choledocholithiasis

Aetiology/pathophysiology/pathology

There are three main types of stone: cholesterol, black pigment (occur in chronic haemolytic disease) and brown pigment stones (associated with infections in the biliary tree). They are almost always found in the gallbladder, and if they escape are usually confined to the extrahepatic biliary tree. Intrahepatic biliary stones are rare, but seen more frequently in the Far East.

Epidemiology

Overall prevalence is 10%. Incidence increases with age and is twice as high in women as in men.

Clinical presentation

Common

- Asymptomatic (incidental finding on imaging).

- Cholestatic liver function tests: raised alkaline phosphatase (ALP) and γ-glutamyltransferase (GGT).

- Indigestion, particularly exacerbated by fatty foods.

- Biliary colic.

- Acute cholecystitis: fever, right upper guadrant pain and tenderness, jaundice.

- Ascending cholangitis: high fever, rigors, jaundice (Virchow's triad).

- Acute pancreatitis.

Uncommon

- Obstructive jaundice without symptoms.

- Gallstone ileus.

⚠️ Elderly patients with cholangitis and secondary Gram-negative septicaemia commonly present with non-specific symptoms, eg 'off legs'.

Physical signs

Common

There may be no signs, although jaundice may be present with right upper quadrant tenderness. In acute cholecystitis look for Murphy's sign.

Rare

The presence of splenomegaly suggests haemolytic anaemia with secondary pigmented common bile duct (CBD) stones.

Investigations

Blood tests

- FBC and reticulocyte count: an elevated white cell count occurs with cholangitis; macrocytic anaemia and elevated reticulocyte count suggests haemolysis.

- Liver biochemistry: classically elevated bilirubin and ALP/GGT; rarely in acute biliary obstruction, aspartate transaminase (AST)/ alanine transaminase (ALT) may be >1000 U/L.

Ultrasound

The preferred investigation for detecting stones in the gallbladder, but remember that the sensitivity for stones in the CBD is only 70% and the only sign may be duct dilatation.

⚠️ The CBD may not be dilated on ultrasound in incomplete biliary obstruction.

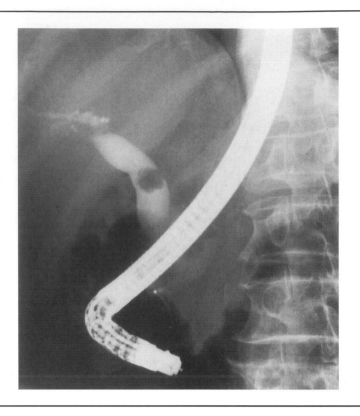

▲ **Fig. 38** ERCP showing a stone in the CBD.

Endoscopic retrograde cholangiopancreatography

Endoscopic retrograde cholangiopancreatography (ERCP) can both confirm that a stone is causing biliary obstruction (Fig. 38) and be employed therapeutically to remove stones. It will also identify any distal CBD stricture, benign or malignant, that may have resulted in proximal stone formation. However, ERCP does carry significant risks and so magnetic resonance cholangiopancreatography (MRCP) (see below) should be considered first (if available) in patients who do not require immediate/urgent therapeutic intervention or if there is diagnostic uncertainty.

Magnetic resonance cholangiopancreatography

This is a non-invasive method of imaging the CBD and pancreatic duct without the need for contrast and therefore has far fewer risks than ERCP. It can be used to detect CBD stones and strictures (see Fig. 24), and consequently ERCP should be considered a therapeutic procedure and should not be performed solely for diagnosis in centres where MRCP is available.

Differential diagnosis

Other causes of biliary obstruction such as tumour or congenital abnormalities such as choledochal cysts.

Treatment

Emergency

Emergency early ERCP (within 72 hours) with removal of CBD stones is indicated in patients with acute pancreatitis associated with obstructive jaundice (see Section 1.4.5). An alternative approach is laparoscopic exploration of the

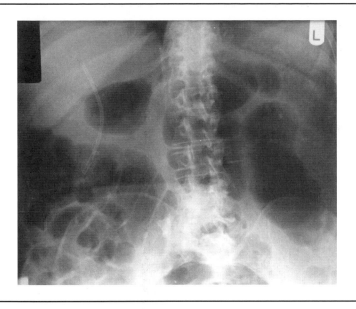

▲ **Fig. 39** Plain abdominal radiograph showing a plastic stent within the CBD.

CBD with stone extraction and cholecystectomy: this may have less morbidity and mortality than ERCP but is not widely available.

Short-term

Endoscopic removal of stones
A sphincterotomy or balloon sphincteroplasty (cutting or dilating the sphincter of Oddi with a balloon) is performed and the CBD trawled with either a balloon or basket to remove the stones. The sphincterotomy allows any retained material to pass. There is a significant risk of acute pancreatitis, bleeding or duodenal perforation, with a 0.5–1% mortality. Larger stones may require crushing with a mechanical lithotriptor or, alternatively, a stent can be inserted to allow bile drainage and a further attempt at removal at a later date. Stenting often causes the stones to shrink over time. Occasionally a nasobiliary drain is required to provide temporary biliary decompression.

Long-term
Interval laparoscopic cholecystectomy in patients for whom surgery is appropriate. In those who are not surgical candidates, and when it is not possible to remove large stones endoscopically, a CBD stent can be left in the bile duct to provide adequate biliary drainage (Fig. 39). This will usually block within 3–12 months and hence most patients are brought back for repeat ERCP and stent exchange every 3–6 months.

Complications
Cholangitis and secondary septicaemia are common. Prolonged asymptomatic biliary obstruction can rarely lead to secondary biliary cirrhosis.

Prognosis
Good if CBD stones are removed.

Disease associations

- Haemolytic anaemia (eg sickle cell) or spherocytosis leading to pigmented large or intrahepatic stones.

- Ileal disease/resection, which interrupts enterohepatic circulation of bile acids.

- *Clonorchis* infection: associated with intrahepatic stones, but exceedingly rare in the UK.

- Total parenteral nutrition: associated with sludge and stones.

FURTHER READING

Beckingham IJ. ABC of diseases of liver, pancreas and biliary system: gallstone disease. *BMJ* 2001; 322: 91–4.

Johnson CD. ABC of the upper gastrointestinal tract: upper abdominal pain – gall bladder. *BMJ* 2001; 323: 1170–3.

Martin DJ, Vernon DR and Toouli J. Surgical versus endoscopic treatment of bile duct stones. *Cochrane Database Syst Rev* 2006; (2): CD003327.

2.5.2 Primary biliary cirrhosis

Aetiology/pathophysiology/ pathology
Primary biliary cirrhosis (PBC) is a disease of unknown aetiology leading to progressive destruction of small intrahepatic bile ducts and eventually to liver cirrhosis and failure. It is thought to be immune mediated as there is a predominantly T-cell infiltration in the liver. It is characterised by female predominance and serum autoantibodies to mitochondrial antigens, most typically targeting the E2 component of the pyruvate dehydrogenase complex (PDC-E2) that lies on the inner mitochondrial membrane. Possible aetiological factors include failure of immune regulation, loss of tolerance, immune complex bile duct damage, and mitochondrial antibodies cross-reacting with bacteria.

Epidemiology
Females account for 90% of cases and most present between the ages

of 40 and 60 years. Prevalence is 25 per 100,000 in women >18 years.

Clinical presentation

Common

- Asymptomatic (diagnosed as a result of investigation for abnormal liver function tests).
- Itching.
- Lethargy.

Uncommon

- Jaundice.
- Haematemesis (from varices).
- Abdominal distension (ascites).
- Confusion (hepatic encephalopathy).
- Hepatocellular carcinoma.

Physical signs

Common

Initially none, subsequently pigmentation, xanthelasma, hepatomegaly, scratch marks.

Uncommon

Late signs of portal hypertension (ascites and hepatic encephalopathy).

Investigations

Liver biochemistry

High alkaline phosphatase and mild increase in alanine transaminase. Rising bilirubin is a marker of poor prognosis. Falling albumin and rising prothrombin time only occur at a very late stage in the disease as it is a biliary cirrhosis.

> The level of alkaline phosphatase does not correlate with the extent of liver disease: insidious progression to cirrhosis may occur without significant changes in liver blood tests.

Anti-mitochondrial antibody

This is present in 95% of cases and is specific for PBC. Individuals with anti-mitochondrial antibody (AMA) and normal liver histology will eventually develop PBC. Patients with AMA-negative biopsy-proven PBC, although rare, behave in the same clinical manner as AMA-positive patients. Anti-nuclear antibodies and/or smooth muscle antibodies are more frequently positive in AMA-negative PBC.

> Non-E2 AMA positivity can be seen in syphilis, systemic lupus erythematosus and other autoimmune diseases.

Immunoglobulins

IgM is often high.

Liver biopsy

The histology is of lymphoid aggregates and granuloma in portal tracts, with bile duct damage and eventually bile duct loss. Progressive fibrosis results in biliary cirrhosis (Fig. 40). Note, however, that liver biopsy is not essential to make the diagnosis of PBC in a patient who has high-titre E2 AMA and typical symptoms and biochemical abnormalities.

> In PBC the changes in the liver are focal so a liver biopsy is not useful for staging liver disease. Furthermore, diagnosis does not usually require liver biopsy because of the specificity of AMA for this disease.

Differential diagnosis

- Large bile duct obstruction.
- Sclerosing cholangitis.

- Other causes of intrahepatic cholestasis (drugs, sepsis, total parenteral nutrition).

Treatment

Short-term

Ursodeoxycholic acid Its role is controversial but it appears to delay time to transplantation and death in late-stage disease. It may improve itching. Treatment at a dose of 10–15 mg/kg should be directed to symptomatic patients.

Other immunosuppressives Steroids, azathioprine, ciclosporin and methotrexate have not convincingly been shown to be effective.

Itching Responds to colestyramine. If persistent, other drugs worth trying include rifampicin, benzodiazepines, ondansetron, serotonin antagonists and naltrexone (opiate antagonist).

Long-term

Liver transplantation Patients who develop signs of decompensated liver disease or in whom bilirubin is greater than 100 µmol/L should be referred to a liver unit if appropriate. Recurrence in hepatic grafts occurs, but this does not have an adverse effect on outcome in the first 5–10 years.

Complications

Osteoporosis and portal hypertension are common in late disease. Osteomalacia and deficiencies of other fat-soluble vitamins are rare.

Prognosis

Variable and unpredictable. Some asymptomatic patients may have a normal life expectancy. Symptoms generally develop within 2–7 years, with subsequent life expectancy varying from 2 to 10 years.

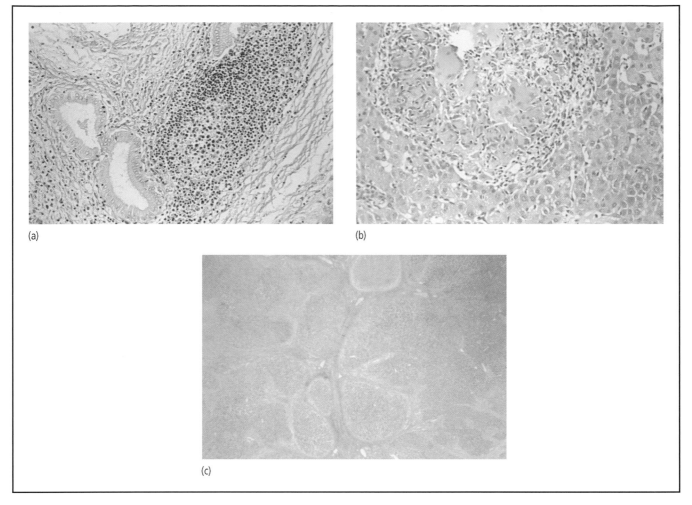

▲ **Fig. 40** Liver biopsy of a patient with primary biliary cirrhosis showing (a) portal tract with lymphocytic infiltration and loss of bile ducts, (b) granuloma and (c) progression to biliary cirrhosis.

Disease associations

Other autoimmune conditions: rheumatoid arthritis, CREST syndrome (*c*alcinosis, *R*aynaud's disease, *e*sophagus (hypomotility), *s*clerodactyly, *t*elangiectasia), hypothyroidism, sicca syndrome (dry mouth and eyes) and coeliac disease.

FURTHER READING

Charatcharoenwitthaya P and Lindor KD. Current concepts in the pathogenesis of primary biliary cirrhosis. *Ann. Hepatol.* 2005; 4: 161–75.

Kaplan MM and Gershwin ME. Primary biliary cirrhosis. *N. Engl. J. Med.* 2005; 353: 1261–73.

2.5.3 Primary sclerosing cholangitis

Aetiology/pathophysiology/pathology

There is diffuse inflammation and fibrosis involving the whole of the biliary tree, eventually leading to obliteration of bile ducts and biliary cirrhosis with portal hypertension. The disease usually involves the intrahepatic ducts alone, but there may also be involvement of the extrahepatic ducts and occasionally the disease is limited to these. The aetiology is unknown, but the disease is probably immunologically mediated. Primary sclerosing cholangitis (PSC) is strongly associated with coexisting inflammatory bowel disease, especially ulcerative colitis, and also with HLA-DR3. Antibodies to perinuclear antineutrophil cytoplasmic antibody are non-specific but seen in 60–80% of cases.

Epidemiology

Prevalence is 6 per 100,000: 70% are male and the average age at diagnosis is 40 years.

Clinical presentation

Fatigue, intermittent jaundice, pruritus, right upper quadrant pain, or no symptoms but abnormal liver biochemistry (often noted in patients with ulcerative colitis or Crohn's disease).

Physical signs

There are no signs in about 50% of symptomatic patients. Jaundice and hepatomegaly or splenomegaly may be present.

Investigations

Liver biochemistry

High alkaline phosphatase/γ-glutamyltransferase. Mild elevations in serum transaminases (aspartate transaminase/alanine transaminase). Bilirubin may be raised. A low albumin and raised prothrombin time are only found in late-stage disease (biliary cirrhosis).

Cholangiography

Percutaneous transhepatic cholangiography or ERCP show multiple irregular stricturing and dilatation (beading) of intrahepatic ducts (Fig. 41), with or without extrahepatic stricture.

Liver biopsy

May be normal. Periductal 'onion skin' fibrosis and inflammation with expansion of portal tracts, bile duct proliferation and portal oedema. Late progressive fibrosis with loss of bile ducts (Fig. 42).

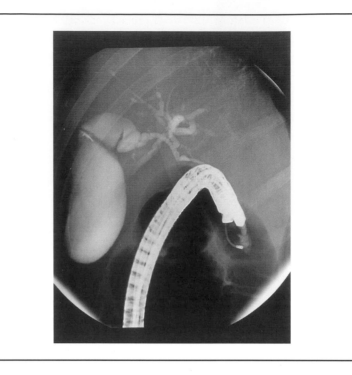

▲**Fig. 41** ERCP showing classical beading of the intrahepatic bile ducts in PSC.

Differential diagnosis

- Secondary sclerosing cholangitis due to cytomegalovirus or *Cryptosporidium* infection in AIDS.

- Previous bile duct surgery.

- Bile duct stones causing cholangitis.

- Post liver transplant recurrent PSC is hard to distinguish from biliary stricturing secondary to hepatic arterial ischaemia.

Treatment

There is no curative therapy.

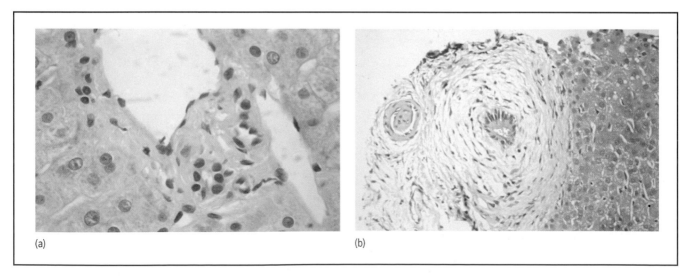

(a)

(b)

▲**Fig. 42** Liver biopsy showing (a) normal portal tract (bile duct, hepatic artery and portal vein) and (b) periductal sclerosis, 'onion skin' fibrosis typical of PSC.

Management of complications

Antibiotics (eg oral ciprofloxacin, which is excreted in bile) for cholangitis. Well-defined extrahepatic biliary strictures can be stented or balloon dilated at ERCP.

Ursodeoxycholic acid

Improves liver biochemistry but probably has no effect on histology or survival. Steroids, azathioprine, methotrexate and ciclosporin have not been shown to have any effect on disease outcome.

Liver transplantation

Indicated for end-stage biliary cirrhosis. Cholangiocarcinoma is a contraindication.

Complications

These include cholangitis, common bile duct or intrahepatic stones, extrahepatic biliary strictures, biliary cirrhosis with portal hypertension, cholangiocarcinoma (occurs in 10–30%, more commonly if the patient has ulcerative colitis) and colorectal carcinoma (25% lifetime risk, especially if the patient has ulcerative colitis). Most of these complications present as increasing jaundice.

> ⚠ It can be difficult to differentiate a benign biliary stricture from a cholangiocarcinoma, even after cholangiography and cytology of brushings from the stricture.

Prognosis

This is variable. In symptomatic patients the median survival from presentation to death or transplantation is 12 years; 75% of asymptomatic patients are alive at 15 years.

Disease associations

Between 5 and 10% of patients with ulcerative colitis and 1% of those with Crohn's disease develop PSC. Up to 70% of patients with PSC will have clinical or histological evidence of ulcerative colitis. The colitis may pre-date the diagnosis of PSC or present many years later.

FURTHER READING

Maggs JR and Chapman RW. Sclerosing cholangitis. *Curr. Opin. Gastroenterol.* 2007; 23: 310–16.

– – – – – – – – – – – – – – – – – –

Olsson R, Boberg KM, de Muckadell OS, *et al.* High-dose ursodeoxycholic acid in primary sclerosing cholangitis: a 5-year multicenter, randomized, controlled study. *Gastroenterology* 2005; 129: 1464–72.

2.5.4 Intrahepatic cholestasis

Cholestasis is defined as an impairment of bile secretion due to intrahepatic or extrahepatic causes. Any disease which leads to failure of synthesis or decreased excretion of bile acids within the liver can result in cholestasis. In addition to intrinsic liver diseases, intrahepatic cholestasis is notable in sepsis, with certain drugs (eg flucloxacillin), following prolonged total parenteral nutrition (TPN), during pregnancy and in a few rare genetic diseases.

Sepsis

Jaundice associated with cholestatic liver biochemistry (elevated alkaline phosphatase and γ-glutamyltransferase) is common in patients with extrabiliary bacterial infections, particularly on the intensive care unit. Differential diagnosis is from cholestasis due to TPN, gallstones and drugs. Treatment is of the underlying condition.

Pregnancy

Intrahepatic cholestasis of pregnancy (ICP) affects about 0.7% of pregnancies in the UK and is associated with prematurity, fetal distress and intrauterine death. It is characterised by pruritus, mostly in the third trimester, and diagnosis is based on the presence of itch in association with elevated levels of serum bile acids and in the absence of other skin diseases. Current medical management is with ursodeoxycholic acid, a hydrophilic bile acid that alters the composition of the bile acid pool in maternal blood. When ICP is diagnosed, ursodeoxycholic acid coupled with close maternal–fetal surveillance is indicated.

Inherited

Progressive familial intrahepatic cholestasis (PFIC) and benign recurrent intrahepatic cholestasis (BRIC) are rare hereditary disorders: patients with PFIC suffer from chronic cholestasis and develop liver fibrosis; patients with BRIC experience intermittent attacks of cholestasis that resolve spontaneously.

2.5.5 Cholangiocarcinoma

Aetiology/pathophysiology/pathology

Chronic inflammation and bile duct stasis are associated with increased risk of developing cholangiocarcinoma, which is a malignant adenocarcinoma of the biliary tree with three main distributions.

1. Intrahepatic or peripheral tumours arising from bile ducts within the liver, usually mass lesions.

2. Extrahepatic tumours that are classified as proximal (near the

liver), intermediate or distal (near the pancreas).

3. Klatskin tumour, which arises at the bifurcation of the common hepatic duct, leading to obstruction of both left and right hepatic ducts.

Epidemiology

Cholangiocarcinomas comprise 5–10% of malignant hepatic tumours and are more common with increasing age (most patients >60 years). The incidence is increasing in the Western world (cause unknown). Intrahepatic cholangiocarcinoma may be mistaken for a liver mass and therefore be under-reported.

Clinical presentation

The patient is often asymptomatic until a late stage, when symptoms include biliary obstruction, fever, weight loss and vague abdominal pain. Some patients describe itching before jaundice becomes clinically apparent.

Physical signs

- Jaundice, with or without hepatomegaly.

- Weight loss.

- Biliary obstruction is usually proximal to the cystic duct, so the gallbladder is not usually palpable (negative Courvoisier's sign).

Investigations

Liver biochemistry

Elevated bilirubin/alkaline phosphatase and γ-glutamyltransferase.

Tumour markers

CA19-9 rises, but does so in many causes of jaundice (benign and malignant) giving a low sensitivity

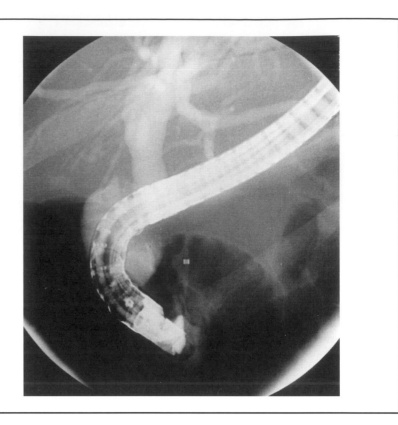

▲ **Fig. 43** ERCP showing a cholangiocarcinoma with dilatation of the CBD above the stricture.

and specificity, so it should not be used diagnostically, although it may be helpful in assessing response to therapy. Alpha-fetoprotein levels will not usually be raised, which can help to differentiate intrahepatic cholangiocarcinomas from hepatocellular carcinoma.

Ultrasound/CT

Ultrasound detects dilated ducts, mass in pancreatic head (carcinoma) and level of obstruction. CT scanning adds little in these patients unless looking for distant metastases.

Endoscopic retrograde cholangiopancreatography

This is usually the definitive test and is both diagnostic and potentially therapeutic (Fig. 43). The sensitivity of cytology of brushing from the stricture is about 50–70%.

Percutaneous transhepatic cholangiography

In the presence of a lower common bile duct (CBD) stricture it may not be possible to cannulate the papilla endoscopically and the biliary tree has to be accessed percutaneously using percutaneous transhepatic cholangiography (PTC) (Fig. 44). PTC is also particularly useful in patients with proximal strictures or Klatskin tumours.

Endoscopic ultrasound

Has been used to take tissue samples by fine-needle aspiration. The use of miniprobes allows further assessment of biliary strictures by intraductal ultrasound in some centres.

Differential diagnosis

Extrahepatic tumours must be differentiated from benign strictures, eg chronic pancreatitis,

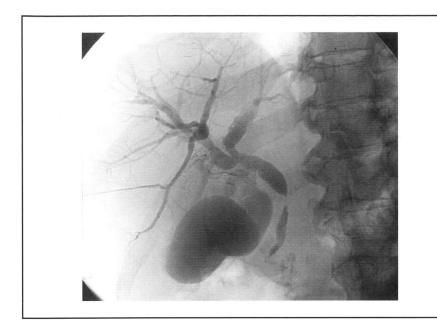

▲**Fig. 44** PTC showing a stricture in the CBD.

primary sclerosing cholangitis. Intrahepatic tumours must be differentiated from hepatic lesions, eg metastases and hepatocellular carcinoma.

Treatment

Short-term

Relief of biliary obstruction with a stent placed percutaneously (Fig. 45)

or endoscopically (Fig. 46) is the mainstay of treatment for most patients. Different types of stent can be employed, selection depending on the predicted survival of the patient: metal self-expanding stents remain patent for longer than cheaper plastic stents.

⚠️ Metal stents cannot be removed and can make subsequent surgery difficult: it is therefore important to have made the correct diagnosis before inserting one.

Long-term

Surgical resection Appropriate in early disease if no evidence of spread. The procedure depends on the location of the tumour. Distal tumours may be removed by Whipple's procedure, with segmental resection for intrahepatic lesions. Klatskin tumours are almost never

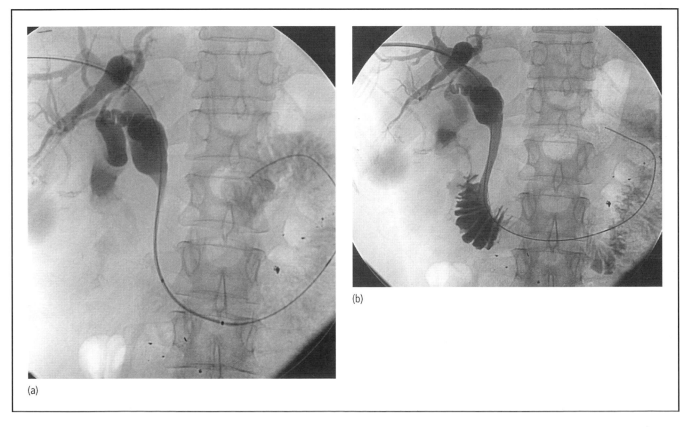

(a) (b)

▲**Fig. 45** (a) A high CBD stricture with dilated intrahepatic ducts above. A percutaneously inserted guidewire can be seen crossing the stricture and passing out of the biliary tree into the duodenum. (b) A metal stent has been placed through the stricture allowing contrast to pass into the duodenum.

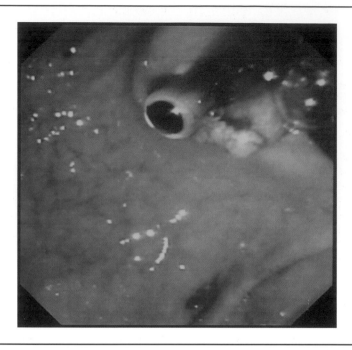

▲ **Fig. 46** Duodenal view of biliary stent showing bile draining freely.

resectable. Roux-en-Y biliary anastomosis may relieve obstruction as a palliative procedure for low CBD cholangiocarcinomas.

Liver transplantation This is contraindicated in a patient with primary sclerosing cholangitis who develops a cholangiocarcinoma due to the high rate of tumour recurrence with immunosuppression.

Complications
Secondary bacterial cholangitis, with or without a blocked stent.

The presence of cholangitis in the presence of a CBD stent usually indicates that the stent is blocked and is an indication for changing it, even if the liver biochemistry improves with treatment of the cholangitis.

Prognosis
This is poor, with an overall survival rate of 40–53% at 1 year and 10–19% at 2 years.

Disease associations
Well-recognised associations are primary sclerosing cholangitis, parasitic infections with liver flukes such as *Clonorchis* and *Opisthorchis* (South-east Asia) and recurrent bacterial cholangitis with hepatolithiasis. Exposure to thorium dioxide (thorotrast), α_1-antitrypsin deficiency and choledochal cysts have also been described in association with cholangiocarcinoma.

FURTHER READING

Khan SA, Davidson BR, Goldin R, *et al.* Guidelines for the diagnosis and treatment of cholangiocarcinoma: consensus document. *Gut* 2002; 51 (Suppl. 6): vi1–vi9. Full text available at http://www.bsg.org.uk/

– – – – – – – – – – – – – – –

Khan SA, Thomas HC, Davidson BR and Taylor-Robinson SD. Cholangiocarcinoma. *Lancet* 2005; 366: 1303–14.

2.6 Infectious diseases

2.6.1 Food poisoning and gastroenteritis
Vomiting and diarrhoea caused by ingestion of contaminated food or water is a common clinical problem. It is common in travellers to areas where pathogens are endemic, or where food and water hygiene is suboptimal. It can also occur in the UK due to pathogens endemic in the food chain and where preparation and storage of food allows organisms or toxins to persist.

Gastrointestinal infections can be caused by viruses (most commonly), bacteria (or their toxins) or protozoa. They present abruptly with diarrhoea and/or vomiting and colicky abdominal pain and are usually self-limiting. The commonest causes in the UK are rotavirus, Norwalk agent, *Campylobacter*, *Salmonella* and *Escherichia coli*.

All cases of 'food poisoning' are notifiable by law.

Stool cultures often fail to grow an organism.

Aetiology/pathophysiology/pathology
Causes of food poisoning and gastroenteritis are shown in Table 37.

Enterotoxins are usually secreted bacterial proteins that act on the intestinal epithelium, or are absorbed into the bloodstream and have systemic effects, eg vibrios and enterotoxigenic *E. coli* toxins can stimulate intestinal secretion.

TABLE 37 CAUSES OF FOOD POISONING AND GASTROENTERITIS

Type of agent	Pathogen	Comment
Viruses	Rotavirus	Outbreaks particularly in young children
	Norwalk	Winter vomiting illness: rapidly spread from person to person
Preformed toxins	*Staphylococcus*	Vomiting and diarrhoea within a few hours of ingesting contaminated food
	Bacillus cereus	Particularly likely to be present in reheated cooked food
Intestinal production of enterotoxins	*Vibrio cholerae*	Usually epidemic outbreaks of severe watery diarrhoea
	Vibrio parahaemolyticus	Vomiting and diarrhoea associated with ingestion of contaminated seafood
Invasive bacterial infection	*E. coli* 0157:H7	Associated with contaminated beef and unpasteurised fruit juices
	Salmonella, *Shigella*, *Campylobacter*	Travellers' diarrhoea and contaminated poultry
Parasites	*Giardia intestinalis*	Water-borne protozoan causing nausea, diarrhoea, flatulence
	Entamoeba histolytica	Cause of dysentery and may cause systemic infection (eg liver abscess)

Enteropathogenic bacteria such as *E. coli*, *Campylobacter*, *Salmonella* and *Shigella* species invade the epithelium, causing ulceration and inflammation. The stool contains blood and leucocytes, and there is a systemic inflammatory response resembling inflammatory bowel disease.

Epidemiology
Worldwide outbreaks, although poorer parts of the world have higher rates of endemic infection.

Clinical presentation
Vomiting and diarrhoea following exposure are the typical features. The main danger of acute gastroenteritis is dehydration and its consequences, which can include life-threatening circulatory collapse, especially in children and in the old and infirm.

Physical signs
Dehydration is the most likely sign. Rectal examination may reveal inflammation and bleeding, particularly if sigmoidoscopy is performed.

Investigation
Stool and vomitus should be collected and analysed for pathogens by microscopy, culture and toxin testing. Food poisoning is a notifiable illness, for obvious public health reasons.

Treatment

Emergency
Dehydration and electrolyte abnormalities should be corrected. In acute gastroenteritis antibiotics have little role, although they may reduce the duration of illness in cases of dysentery.

Complications
Reactive arthritis may develop after a self-limited episode of food poisoning. Guillain–Barré syndrome may follow infection with *Campylobacter* species.

Prevention
Food hygeine and meticulous cooking of potentially contaminated meat and poultry are the key measures.

2.6.2 Bacterial dysentery

Aetiology/pathophysiology/pathology
Infection is spread by consuming contaminated water or food, particularly meat and poultry. Common causes of bacterial dysentery are *Campylobacter jejuni*, *Salmonella* species, *Shigella* species and enteropathogenic *E. coli* strains.

Epidemiology
Travellers to endemic areas in the tropics, subtropics and poor countries with inadequate sanitation and food hygiene practices are most affected. *Salmonella* infection is endemic in poultry in the UK, and undercooked or raw eggs and chicken are a common cause of infection. *E. coli* strain 0157:H7 is endemic in cattle and causes outbreaks associated with ingestion of contaminated beef.

Bacterial dysentery is not only a disease of travellers: *Salmonella* infection is endemic in poultry in the UK and can contaminate the food chain.

Clinical presentation
The incubation period is 3–5 days. Dysentery typically causes severe, cramping abdominal pain and diarrhoea, which may be bloody. There is frequently associated malaise, headache and myalgia. Infection with *E. coli* strain 0157:H7 may be associated with severe renal dysfunction and haemolysis, and may be rapidly fatal. Bacterial dysentery may be indistinguishable

from idiopathic inflammatory bowel disease (IBD) and may occur in patients who already have a diagnosis of IBD.

> Sigmoidoscopic and histological appearances in gastrointestinal infections and idiopathic IBD may be indistinguishable, and the two conditions can also coexist.

Complications

Bacterial dysentery may cause Reiter's syndrome (uveitis or conjunctivitis, urethritis and arthritis). Guillain–Barré syndrome may follow infection with *Campylobacter* species. *Salmonella* infection may become systemic (eg causing osteomyelitis or septic arthritis), and a chronic carrier state associated with colonisation of the biliary tree is sometimes established.

> Infection with *E. coli* strain O157:H7 can follow ingestion of contaminated food, especially beef, and is associated with a severe life-threatening haemolytic–uraemic syndrome.

Treatment

Fluoroquinolones such as ciprofloxacin are usually highly effective. Haemolytic–uraemic syndrome caused by *E. coli* O157:H7 infection requires high-intensity supportive treatment.

2.6.3 Antibiotic-associated diarrhoea

Aetiology/pathophysiology/pathology

Use of antibiotics alters the enteric bacterial population and frequently causes diarrhoea. In some cases this

is caused by overgrowth of enterotoxin-producing *Clostridium difficile*. Most antibiotics are implicated, including clindamycin, with the widespread use of third-generation cephalosporins and broad-spectrum penicillins responsible for many cases.

Clinical presentation

Diarrhoea may be mild, with frequent watery stools, or more severe, with passage of blood and mucus and a marked systemic inflammatory response (fever, tachycardia, hypotension). The most severe consequence of toxigenic *C. difficile* infection, pseudomembranous colitis, may lead to intestinal perforation and is life-threatening.

Investigations

C. difficile can be cultured from the stool and its enterotoxins can be detected by a sensitive and rapid enzyme-linked immunosorbent assay (ELISA). Sigmoidoscopy reveals punctate yellow-white plaques adhering to inflamed mucosa in pseudomembranous colitis.

> *C. difficile* enterotoxin can be detected by a rapid and specific ELISA performed on stool specimens.

Prevention and treatment

Strategies to minimise the use of broad-spectrum antibiotics reduce the incidence of *C. difficile* infection. First-line treatment is with metronidazole, administered orally or parenterally. Relapse is common (up to 30%) and can be treated by vancomycin 125 mg qds orally. Probiotics may reduce the incidence of further relapses.

FURTHER READING

Bricker E, Garg R, Nelson R, *et al.* Antibiotic treatment for *Clostridium difficile*-associated diarrhea in adults. *Cochrane Database Syst Rev* 2005; (1): CD004610.

Hurley BW and Nguyen CC. The spectrum of pseudomembranous enterocolitis and antibiotic-associated diarrhea. *Arch. Intern. Med.* 2002; 162: 2177–84.

2.6.4 Parasitic infestations of the intestine

Aetiology/pathophysiology/pathology

Intestinal parasitic infestations are widespread throughout the world. In the UK the commonest infestations are with *Giardia intestinalis* and *Enterobius vermicularis* (pinworm). Hookworm and roundworm infections may cause chronic diarrhoea, malabsorption, growth retardation and intestinal blood loss.

> Infection with *Giardia intestinalis* and *Enterobius vermicularis* are widespread in the UK.

Clinical presentation

Giardiasis is spread by the fecal–oral route and by ingesting contaminated water. The organism is relatively resistant to chlorine. Infection typically causes nausea and diarrhoea with excessive flatus after an incubation period of 1–4 weeks. Malabsorption may occur, with pale, bulky, offensive stools and weight loss. Symptoms may persist for months.

Pinworm infection is spread by the fecal–oral route from human to human. It is particularly prevalent among children and may cause perianal pruritis as the organisms and eggs are shed.

Investigations

Giardiasis is diagnosed by finding trophozoites in jejunal aspirates or biopsies taken at endoscopy, or cysts in the stool. Pinworms or oocytes might be detected in the stool.

Treatment

Metronidazole or tinidazole are highly effective for giardiasis, while pinworm infections are treated with mebendazole or albendazole. Household contacts should be treated.

2.6.5 Intestinal and liver amoebiasis

Aetiology/pathophysiology/pathology

Entamoeba histolytica is a free-living protozoan that spreads via person-to-person contact and by ingestion of contaminated water or food. It can cause dysentery when localised to the large intestine. The organisms are distributed haematogenously to distant organs, particularly the liver, where they may cause inflammatory masses (amoeboma) and abscesses.

Clinical presentation

The incubation period for amoebic dysentery is 1–4 weeks. Symptoms range from mild diarrhoea to severe bloody diarrhoea (colonic ulceration). Amoebic liver abscess may present many months after infection with abdominal pain, fever and abnormal liver function tests.

Investigations

Dysentery is diagnosed by examination of the stool, which may demonstrate live parasites, or by rectal biopsy or serology. Amoebic abscesses are visualised by imaging,

such as ultrasound, and may require aspiration and microscopy.

Complications

Liver abscesses occur in 1–3% of cases.

Treatment

Metronidazole is effective in treating amoebic dysentery. Liver abscesses should be treated with metronidazole followed by diloxanide to eliminate carriage of the organism.

2.6.6 Intestinal features of HIV infection

Despite progress in treating HIV infection, infection rates are increasing worldwide as well as in the UK. Up to one-third of HIV-positive individuals in the UK may be unaware of their infected status.

Untreated HIV progresses to cause a profound immune deficiency, and with immunodeficiency the gastrointestinal tract may be involved by oropharyngeal and oesophageal candidiasis, cryptosporidiosis, microsporidiosis, atypical mycobacterial infection, tuberculosis, cytomegalovirus and herpesvirus infections. HIV-positive patients may also be at greater risk of enteric pathogens such as amoebiasis and dysentery-causing bacteria.

> **Gastroenteritits caused by unusual organisms, oropharyngeal candidiasis, and severe and persistent herpesvirus infection raise the possibility of HIV infection.**

HIV infection itself may cause an enteropathy, manifest as diarrhoea, malabsorption and weight loss, which histologically has the appearance of partial villous atrophy with crypt hyperplasia and

polymorph infiltration. Depletion of lymphocytes in the gastrointestinal tract is an early feature of HIV infection, and in patients on antiretroviral drug treatment a reservoir of latent virus may persist in gastrointestinal lymphoid tissue.

Co-infection with HIV and hepatitis C or B viruses causes more severe and rapidly progressive liver disease. Antiretroviral drug treatment may cause severe drug-induced hepatitis, hence (for instance) nevirapine should not be used in individuals with a high or normal CD4 count because it can induce a life-threatening hepatitis.

> **HIV and the liver**
> - Chronic viral hepatitis is usually more severe in the presence of HIV co-infection.
> - Antiretroviral drug treatment may cause severe liver disease.

2.7 Inflammatory bowel disease

2.7.1 Crohn's disease

Aetiology/pathophysiology/pathology

The aetiology is unknown, but there is a presumed autoimmune process (association with perinuclear antineutrophil cytoplasmic antibody and antibodies to Baker's yeast). There is a measurable genetic component, with family studies showing 50% concordance in identical twins and linkage studies incriminating a number of loci. There is also a possible association with infectious agents, eg *Mycobacterium paratuberculosis*. There is an increased incidence in cigarette smokers.

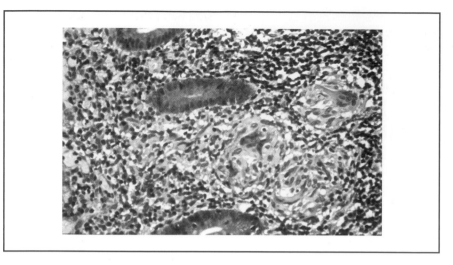

▲**Fig. 47** Histological specimen from Crohn's colitis showing intense inflammation and granuloma.

The characteristic histological features are transmural inflammation with ulceration and granuloma formation (Fig. 47). This may affect any part of the gastrointestinal tract (mouth to anus), but predominantly the terminal ileum, right colon or rectum and perianal region. Affected areas are often separated by normal bowel ('skip lesions'). The process may cause strictures or fistulae to adjacent structures and is usually accompanied by a vigorous systemic response, with raised C-reactive protein (CRP) and erythrocyte sedimentation rate (ESR).

Epidemiology

Incidence is 6–8 per 100,000 and prevalence is 26–56 per 100,000 in northern Europe, the USA and Australia. Slightly more common in females. There is a bimodal age incidence: 15–40 years is most common, with a second peak at around 70 years of age. Ten per cent of patients have a first-degree relative with the disease. The risk for siblings is 30-fold increased compared with the general population. Smoking increases relative risk three-fold.

Clinical presentation

Common

Diarrhoea, abdominal pain and weight loss (often >10% body mass) are all expected, with Crohn's disease the presumed diagnosis in a young patient with this triad. May be associated with general malaise, lassitude, fever and anorexia. A careful history may reveal a lengthy preceding history of bowel upset, a previous diagnosis of irritable bowel syndrome, or previous perianal disease (fissure or abscess).

Rare

Occasionally mistaken for anorexia nervosa.

Physical signs

Common

There may be few physical signs, or the patient may be thin and unwell with clubbing, aphthous ulceration, abdominal tenderness, and perianal skin tags, ulceration or fistulae.

Uncommon

Abdominal mass.

Rare

Fistulae, seronegative arthritis, sacroiliitis, iritis and skin rashes (erythema nodosum, pyoderma gangrenosum).

Investigations

Blood tests

FBC often shows anaemia, which may be normochromic, normocytic (chronic disease) or result from iron, B_{12} or folate deficiency. The platelet count is often high in active disease (regard as an 'inflammatory marker'). Serum inflammatory markers are raised (CRP and ESR). Serum albumin is often low (due to chronic inflammatory disease process, not malnutrition). Vitamin B_{12} may be low due to terminal ileitis.

Other tests

Sigmoidoscopy/colonoscopy can show colonic or ileal inflammation (may be patchy), granulomas on biopsy and is the investigation of choice. Small bowel follow-through can show segmental inflammation, strictures and fistulae (Fig. 48). MRI scanning is particularly useful for assessing complex perianal disease, including fistulae.

> Rectal biopsy in Crohn's disease may show granuloma even when macroscopically normal.

Differential diagnosis

- Ulcerative colitis if colonic involvement.

- Abdominal tuberculosis, particularly if terminal ileal disease and the patient is in an 'at-risk' group.

- Malignancy/intestinal lymphoma.

Treatment

Emergency

Patients who are very ill will require emergency admission to hospital for

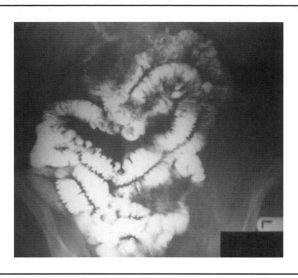

▲**Fig. 48** Barium follow-through showing several tight strictures in the terminal ileum in a patient with Crohn's disease.

resuscitation followed by treatment as described in Sections 1.4.2 and 1.4.4.

Short-term

Corticosteroids In severe disease start hydrocortisone 100 mg iv qid. Following clinical response, or if the attack is less severe, commence oral prednisolone at 30–40 mg daily and taper down by approximately 5 mg per fortnight depending on clinical progress; 70% will be in remission in 3–4 months. Budesonide, a topically acting steroid with high potency and extensive first-pass metabolism, is equivalent to prednisolone in inducing remission in terminal ileal disease and has fewer side effects, but is much more expensive and relapse rates within 1 year are disappointingly high.

5-Aminosalicylic acids These compounds have only marginal benefit in acute disease.

Dietary Elemental and polymeric diets containing low-molecular-weight nutrients may induce remission in up to 70% of patients (particularly in small bowel disease).

They need to be taken cold as a sip feed and may have to be given by nasogastric tube (for 6 weeks).

Other Metronidazole or ciprofloxacin may be useful in treating perianal sepsis, but the evidence for this is not strong.

Long-term

About 50% of Crohn's disease patients will have relapsed 1 year after initial treatment.

5-Aminosalicylic acids Have at best a modest effect in maintaining remission, with the postsurgical subgroup benefiting most.

Azathioprine This immunosuppressant has been shown to induce remission in steroid-resistant and steroid-dependent patients, to reduce relapse rates (including post surgery), and to have steroid-sparing effects. It takes 6–12 weeks to achieve its effects. Side effects include bone marrow suppression, liver dysfunction (dose dependent) and pancreatitis (idiosyncratic). Patients should have FBC checked

weekly for the first month, then monthly for 2 months, and 3-monthly for the duration of treatment.

Methotrexate In those intolerant of, or failing to respond to, azathioprine, methotrexate may be tried. In steroid-dependent patients it has been shown to achieve both remission and withdrawal of steroids in 39% compared with 19% given placebo.

Infliximab This anti-tumour necrosis factor (TNF)-α antibody is established in the treatment of refractory Crohn's disease. It may induce long-term remission in up to 60% of patients and has recently been licensed for maintenance therapy, although it remains very expensive. All patients should have a CXR to exclude previous tuberculosis prior to starting treatment.

Surgery Crohn's patients have a 90% lifetime risk of surgery (Fig. 49). Indications include failed medical therapy, abscesses, fistulae, intestinal obstruction and haemorrhage, and in limited terminal ileal disease it may be considered the treatment of choice. Half will have symptomatic relapse within 10 years following surgery, although up to 80% may have evidence of disease at endoscopy, but not all will require further operations. Strictureplasty may be performed, rather than resection, to preserve small intestinal length.

Complications

Common

Intestinal obstruction Usually subacute. May be due to active disease causing oedema and narrowing, or to chronic fibrotic stricture. The former usually responds to steroids.

97

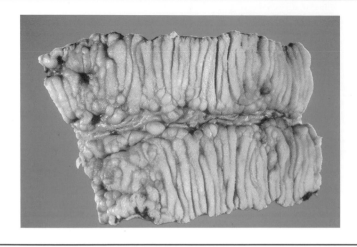

▲ **Fig. 49** Terminal ileum resected from a patient with Crohn's disease showing linear ulceration and pseudopolyps.

> 🔑 Patients with small bowel strictures are advised to maintain a low-fibre diet to avoid food bolus obstruction.

Malabsorption Vitamin B$_{12}$ deficiency and bile salt diarrhoea are caused by terminal ileal disease. Extensive involvement of the small bowel or surgical resections result in generalised malabsorption (short bowel syndrome). Bacterial overgrowth secondary to enteroenteric fistulae or strictures results in fat malabsorption.

Perforations Contained perforations result in abdominal, pelvic and ischiorectal abscesses and require drainage.

Uncommon/rare

- Chronic blood loss causing iron-deficiency anaemia.

- Massive rectal bleeding, almost always secondary to colonic disease.

- Toxic megacolon can occur, but is less common than in ulcerative colitis.

- There is an increased risk of colonic carcinoma in patients with colonic Crohn's disease.

- Free perforation is rare.

Prognosis

Morbidity

Some patients experience considerable morbidity from general ill-health, pain, malnutrition, fistulous disease, abscess formation, repeated surgery or steroid side effects, but most are maintained relatively symptom-free.

Mortality

Overall mortality is twice that for the general population. Those diagnosed with the disease before the age of 20 have more than 10 times the standardised mortality ratio.

Prevention

Cessation of smoking is of benefit in active disease and reduces the risk of relapse.

Disease associations

Weak association with primary sclerosing cholangitis, arthralgia and arthritis; also with HLA-B27.

FURTHER READING

Carter MJ, Lobo AJ and Travis SPL (on behalf of the IBD Section of the British Society of Gastroenterology). Guidelines for the management of inflammatory bowel disease in adults. *Gut* 2004; 53 (Suppl. 5): v1–v16. Full text available at http://www.bsg.org.uk/

- - - - - - - - - - - - - - - - - - - -

Caprilli R, Gassull MA, Escher JC, *et al.* European evidence based consensus on the diagnosis and management of Crohn's disease: special situations. *Gut* 2006; 55 (Suppl. 1): i36–i58.

- - - - - - - - - - - - - - - - - - - -

Stange EF, Travis SPL, Vermiere S, *et al.* European evidence based consensus on the diagnosis and management of Crohn's disease: definitions and diagnosis. *Gut* 2006; 55 (Suppl. 1): i1–i15.

- - - - - - - - - - - - - - - - - - - -

Travis SPL, Stange EF, Lemann M, *et al.* European evidence based consensus on the diagnosis and management of Crohn's disease: current management. *Gut* 2006; 55 (Suppl. 1): i16–i35.

2.7.2 Ulcerative colitis

Aetiology/pathophysiology/pathology

The aetiology is unknown, but there is a presumed autoimmune process with a measurable genetic component (genetic linkages and family studies). Enteric bacterial factors seem to be important. There is a decreased incidence in cigarette smokers.

The histopathological features are of mucosal inflammation only (contrasting with Crohn's disease) with crypt distortion, crypt abscesses and goblet cell depletion (Fig. 50).

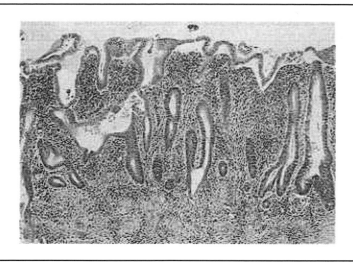

▲**Fig. 50** Histology of ulcerative colitis showing inflammatory infiltrate within the mucosa.

Rectal inflammation is almost universal, but the extent of more proximal disease is variable. Disease is continuous, ie extends from anus to wherever the proximal extent lies, and does not cause fistulae or strictures, but may rarely result in fibrotic narrowing of colon.

Epidemiology
Incidence 10–20 per 100,000. Affects any age group, but most typically youths and young adults.

Clinical presentation
Bloody diarrhoea and general malaise are common. Arthritis and arthralgia, uveitis, skin rashes, abdominal pain and tenesmus are less common. Toxic megacolon is rare.

Physical signs

Common
There may be few physical signs, but the patient may be thin and unwell with aphthous ulceration, abdominal tenderness, blood on rectal examination, and mucopus on rigid sigmoidoscopy.

Uncommon
Toxic megacolon, arthritis, iritis and skin rashes (erythema nodosum, pyoderma gangrenosum).

Investigations/staging
Serum inflammatory markers are markedly raised in severe disease but may be normal in proctitis or mild disease. Stool culture and microscopy are required to exclude infectious diarrhoea, including *Clostridium difficile*.

Plain abdominal radiograph
May show proximal faecal loading. Mucosal oedema and ulcers may be detected, and in severe disease there can be colonic dilatation (toxic megacolon).

Barium enema
This may confirm findings on the plain abdominal radiograph, but its use is limited and should be avoided in severe disease due to the risk of perforation (Fig. 51).

Colonoscopy
The investigation of choice in ulcerative colitis: may show inflammation extending from the rectum to the proximal extent of disease (Fig. 52). In severe disease this should be limited to flexible sigmoidoscopy due to the increased risk of perforation.

Differential diagnosis
Common differential diagnoses include Crohn's colitis, infectious colitis (bacterial, amoebic, viral, eg cytomegalovirus in immunosuppressed patients), NSAID-induced colitis, and microscopic colitis.

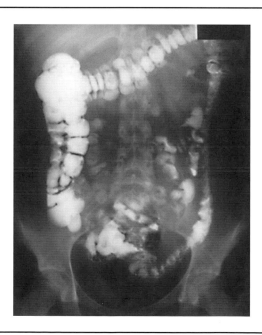

▲**Fig. 51** Barium enema showing ulcerative colitis extending to the splenic flexure.

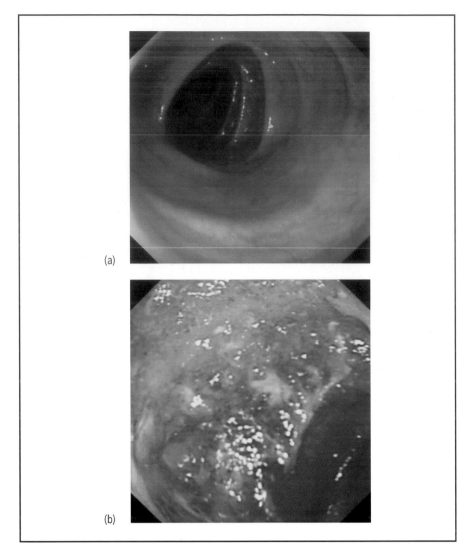

(a)

(b)

▲ **Fig. 52** Endoscopic appearance of (**a**) normal colon and (**b**) inflamed colon.

Treatment

Emergency

Patients who are very ill will require emergency admission to hospital for resuscitation followed by treatment as described in Sections 1.4.2 and 1.4.4.

Short-term

In mild to moderate disease, high-dose 5-aminosalicylic acid compounds (4 g/day) may induce remission. The addition of topical preparations can result in more rapid resolution of rectal bleeding and are the first-line treatment of choice in proctitis and colitis not extending beyond the splenic flexure. In more severe disease, or where 5-aminosalicylic acid compounds are ineffective, steroids may be used, eg prednisolone 30–40 mg/day, reduced by 5 mg every 1–2 weeks. Intravenous ciclosporin may have a role to play in severe colitis, but this remains controversial due to potential side effects and high long-term failure rates.

Long-term

5-Aminosalicylic acid compounds can maintain remission in most patients. In patients who have frequent relapses or become steroid dependent, immunosuppression with azathioprine (target dose 2–2.5 mg/kg) is recommended. Panproctocolectomy is curative. Patients may opt for a permanent ileostomy or formation of a neorectum using a loop of ileum (pouch).

Complications

Common complications include malnutrition, steroid-induced side effects, arthralgias, arthritis, skin rash. Less common are uveitis, toxic megacolon and perforation or sepsis. Malignancy (colorectal carcinoma) is rare.

> Because of the increased risk of colorectal cancer, it is now recommended that all patients with ulcerative colitis undergo surveillance colonoscopy every 3 years after 10 years, every 2 years after 20 years, and yearly from 30 years. However, the use of regular 5-aminosalicylic acid compounds may reduce the risk to near that of the normal population.

Prognosis

Morbidity

About 25% of patients experience only one attack, 40% are in remission in any one year, and a minority have unremitting disease. About 30% of patients ultimately undergo colectomy. The longer a patient remains in remission, the better the chance of remaining in remission.

Mortality

Overall mortality is not increased compared with healthy controls, possibly due to a lower incidence of smoking.

Prevention

Secondary prevention is with 5-aminosalicylic acid compounds and azathioprine.

Disease associations

Primary sclerosing cholangitis.

FURTHER READING

Carter MJ, Lobo AJ and Travis SPL (on behalf of the IBD Section of the British Society of Gastroenterology). Guidelines for the management of inflammatory bowel disease in adults. *Gut* 2004; 53 (Suppl. 5): v1–v16. Full text available at http://www.bsg.org.uk/

– – – – – – – – – – – – – – – –

Podolsky DK. Inflammatory bowel disease. *N. Engl. J. Med.* 2002; 347: 417–29.

– – – – – – – – – – – – – – – –

Stein RB and Hanauer SB. Medical therapy for inflammatory bowel disease. *Gastroenterol. Clin. North Am.* 1999; 28: 297–321.

2.7.3 Microscopic colitis

Aetiology/pathophysiology/ pathology

The aetiology of microscopic colitis is not known, but there is a recognised association with coeliac disease, raising the possiblity of gluten sensitivity as an aetiological factor, and also an association with the use of NSAIDs. Colonoscopy is macroscopically normal, but histology may show a marked rise in intraepithelial lymphocytes (lymphocytic colitis) or a thick subepithelial collagen layer (collagenous colitis).

Epidemiology

Occurs typically in middle-aged and elderly women. More common than originally thought, with combined incidence of about 8–10 per 100,000.

Clinical presentation

Most commonly with persistent watery diarrhoea. Less commonly weight loss and abdominal pain may be seen in cases with coexisting coeliac disease.

Physical signs

There are usually no abnormal physical signs. Rigid sigmoidoscopy is typically normal.

Investigations/staging

Serum inflammatory markers, macroscopic appearance at colonoscopy and barium enema are usually normal. Coeliac antibodies should be checked and duodenal biopsies arranged if these are positive. Microscopic changes in the colon (raised intraepithelial lymphocytes or a thick subendothelial collagen band) are diagnostic, but there may be a 40% false-negative rate if only left-sided biopsies are taken, so samples should also be taken from the ascending colon.

Differential diagnosis

Other cause of chronic diarrhoea (see Section 1.1.3).

Treatment

The condition may be self-limiting. Antidiarrhoeal agents (eg loperamide) may be sufficient in mild disease. 5-Aminosalicylic acid compounds may be of benefit in mild to moderate disease, with improvement seen in up to 50% of cases. Bismuth subsalicylate has been advocated, but trial data are limited and there remain concerns over potential toxic side effects. In resistant cases budesonide (a potent corticosteroid with high first-pass metabolism and thus low systemic side-effect profile) seems to be more efficacious than conventional corticosteroid therapy with prednisolone. Colestyramine may be of value, with some case series reporting incidence of concomitant bile salt malabsorption as high as 60%. There are no good data for any of the mentioned drugs in maintenance of remission.

Prognosis

Most patients suffer repeated relapses.

Disease associations

Arthritis, thyroiditis, diabetes, coeliac disease.

FURTHER READING

Chande N, McDonald JW and MacDonald JK. Interventions for treating lymphocytic colitis. *Cochrane Database Syst Rev* 2007; Jan 24: CD006096.

– – – – – – – – – – – – – – – –

Stroehlein R. Microscopic colitis. *Curr. Opin. Gastroenterol.* 2004; 20: 27–31.

2.8 Functional bowel disorders

There are a range of functional bowel disorders (Table 38). The rest of this section concentrates on the commonest of these, irritable bowel syndrome.

Aetiology/pathophysiology/ pathology

The hallmark of the functional gastrointestinal disorders is altered (usually increased) visceral pain sensitivity. This may be associated with increased release of 5-hydroxytryptamine (5HT, serotonin) from enterochromaffin cells in the gut, but central (psychosocial, neurohumoral) factors may be important, and it has also been suggested that alterations in the intestinal bacterial flora may be involved. This is supported by the high incidence of patients presenting with irritable bowel syndrome following culture-positive gastroenteritis, use of broad-spectrum antibiotics or pelvic surgery. The role of stress is uncertain, but there is a higher

TABLE 38 THE FUNCTIONAL BOWEL DISORDERS

Classification	Examples
Oesophageal disorders	Globus Functional heartburn Functional dysphagia
Gastroduodenal disorders	Functional dyspepsia Functional vomiting
Bowel disorders	Irritable bowel syndrome Functional constipation Functional diarrhoea Functional abdominal pain
Biliary disorders	Sphincter of Oddi dysfunction
Anorectal disorders	Functional faecal incontinence Proctalgia fugax Functional paediatric disorders

incidence of psychological disorders in those who seek medical advice.

Epidemiology

The prevalence of the functional bowel disorders depends entirely on definition. It is estimated that only 10–50% of patients with functional gut symptoms consult medical practitioners, yet this represents as much as 5% of all general practice consultations in the UK and up to 40% of gastroenterology referrals. There is a female to male predominance of 2–3:1. About 75% of patients diagnosed with irritable bowel syndrome will continue to have chronic disease.

Clinical presentation

Common

The agreed definition of irritable bowel syndrome is as follows: 'At least 12 weeks, which need not be consecutive, in the preceding 12 months of abdominal discomfort or pain that has two of the following three features: relieved with defecation; and/or onset associated with a change in frequency of stool; and/or onset associated with a change in form (appearance) of stool.'

Symptoms that cumulatively support the diagnosis of irritable bowel syndrome include abnormal stool frequency (more than three motions per day or less than three motions per week); abnormal stool form; abnormal stool passage (urgency, straining or incomplete evacuation); passage of mucus; bloating or a feeling of abdominal distension.

> There are some clinical features that should not be attributed to a functional cause without careful further investigation, including:
>
> - dysphagia;
> - anorexia and/or weight loss;
> - mouth ulcers;
> - nocturnal diarrhoea;
> - rectal bleeding.

Physical signs

There are no characteristic physical signs.

Investigation

The extent of clinical investigation must be tailored to the individual patient. A detailed history (including a good dietary history) is central to both the correct clinical diagnosis and subsequent management. Investigations depend largely on the patient's particular symptom complex. A recommended screening panel would include FBC, erythrocyte sedimentation rate, thyroid function tests and coeliac antibodies. Where appropriate consider stool cultures. Patients aged over 50 years presenting with altered bowel habit should have a colonoscopy.

Differential diagnosis

The following should always be considered: coeliac disease, hypolactasia, inflammatory bowel disease, giardiasis, depressive illness, gastrointestinal malignancy and thyroid disease (hyperthyroidism and hypothyroidism). The diffential diagnosis for chronic diarrhoea is described in Section 1.1.3.

Treatment

> The most important part of the management is to listen to the patient: after a thorough history and physical examination the 'qualified reassurance' of being told that there is no objective evidence of physical disease may be sufficient to lead to an improvement in symptoms (or at least the resulting concern).

The treatment of irritable bowel syndrome sufferers is often disappointing but should be tailored to the predominant symptoms of the patient (Table 39).

Prognosis

Most patients will continue to have intermittent gastrointestinal symptoms and some may develop more overt psychiatric problems. Mortality is not increased.

FURTHER READING

Carter MJ, Lobo AJ and Travis SPL (on behalf of the IBD Section of the British Society of Gastroenterology). Guidelines for the management of inflammatory bowel disease in adults. *Gut* 2004; 53 (Suppl. 5): v1–v16. Full text available at http://www.bsg.org.uk/

Kennedy T, Rubin G and Jones R. Irritable bowel syndrome. *Clin. Evid.* 2004; 11: 615–25.

Mertz HR. Irritable bowel syndrome. *N. Engl. J. Med.* 2003; 349: 2136–46.

TABLE 39 TREATMENTS FOR PATIENTS WITH IRRITABLE BOWEL SYNDROME

Main symptom	Treatments
Diarrhoea	Dietary exclusion: common problem foods include wheat, dairy and eggs; many patients benefit from a low-fibre diet and find their symptoms worsen with increase in dietary fibre Antidiarrhoeals (loperamide, diphenoxylate) $5HT_3$ antagonists, eg alosteron, but concern remains over the association with ischaemic colitis Amitriptyline
Constipation	Fibre supplementation: this may be achieved by dietary means, but may result in increased pain or bloating; non-fermentable bulking agents (eg Normacol) may be more efficacious Laxatives: stimulant laxatives (eg senakot) are not recommended for long-term use; osmotic laxatives, eg Movicol (macrogols) or other polyethylene glycol-based preparations, are most effective Biofeedback: particularly if straining is a predominant symptom; retrains individuals to defecate normally
Pain/bloating	Anitcholinergics (eg mebeverine, alverine): reduce bowel spasm Amitriptyline: has anticholinergic effects and works on serotonin pathway; effective at small (10–25 mg) doses independently from presence of depressive symptoms, but side-effect profile may limit use. SSRIs: act on serotonin pathway; fewer side effects than amitriptyline but data less convincing Hypnotherapy

SSRIs, selective serotonin reuptake inhibitors.

2.9 Large bowel disorders

Colorectal cancer remains a major cause of death worldwide. It commonly presents at an advanced stage with complications such as colonic obstruction or perforation, but recognition that most cancers arise within adenomatous polyps of the colon (Fig. 53) has led to a greater emphasis on early diagnosis.

2.9.1 Adenomatous polyps of the colon

Aetiology/pathophysiology/pathology

These are benign neoplastic polyps. The cause is uncertain, but may be related to genetic abnormalities or diet. Although slow-growing they may develop malignant potential, especially if greater than 1 cm in diameter or if they demonstrate high-grade dysplasia on microscopy.

Clinical presentation

Most commonly an incidental finding at colonoscopy, but sometimes can present with iron-deficiency anaemia and/or rectal bleeding.

Polyps found during colonoscopy for investigation of iron-deficieny anaemia may not be the cause but merely an incidental finding.

Differential diagnosis

Not all colonic polyps carry a significantly increased risk of colorectal cancer.

Hyperplastic polyps

These are diminutive polyps, usually less than 5 mm in diameter, found in the distal colon and rectum. They are not neoplastic and carry no significant risk of colorectal cancer. 'Hyperplastic polyps' found beyond the splenic flexure should be followed up as they may be serrated adenomas, which do have malignant potential.

Hamartomatous polyps

These are associated with Peutz–Jeghers syndrome, and although they are not themselves neoplastic, there is an increased risk of gastrointestinal tumours in these patients.

Inflammatory pseudopolyps

Representing islands of regenerative mucosa in a chronically inflamed bowel, these are seen in Crohn's disease and ulcerative colitis. They carry no malignant potential.

Treatment

Colonoscopic polypectomy is recommended for all adenomatous polyps. Further surveillance for these patients is discussed in Section 2.9.2.

Complications
Colorectal carcinoma.

FURTHER READING

Levine JS and Ahnen DJ. Clinical practice: adenomatous polyps of the colon. *N. Engl. J. Med.* 2006; 355: 2551–7.

2.9.2 Colorectal carcinoma

Colorectal cancer is a major public health problem in the developed world: increasing efforts are being directed towards early identification of the condition in individuals considered to be at risk.

Aetiology/pathophysiology/ pathology
There are several conditions that are recognised to predispose to colorectal cancer.

Adenomatous polyps of the colon
Tubulovillous adenomas carry an increased risk of colorectal cancer. It is generally felt that colorectal cancer usually develops in pre-existing adenomatous polyps in the colon (Fig. 53).

Ulcerative colitis
Patients with a 10-year history of colitis extending proximal to the splenic flexure are at increased risk of colorectal carcinoma. They should be offered surveillance colonoscopy with random pancolonic biopsies to detect dysplastic change (see Prevention).

Family history
There is a family history in 14% of new cases of colorectal cancer. Lifetime risk can be calculated based on family history and surveillance recommended accordingly (Table 40).

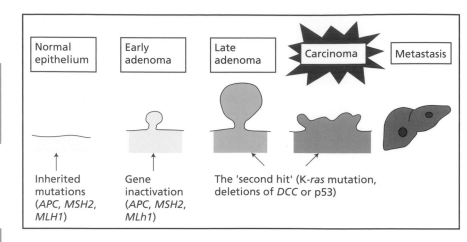

▲**Fig. 53** The colonic adenoma–carcinoma sequence. *DCC* (deleted in colon cancer), *APC*, *MLH1* and *MSH2* are genes.

Familial cancer syndromes
There are some rare but important hereditary cancer syndromes.

- Familial adenomatous polyposis (FAP): autosomal dominant; hundreds of adenomatous polyps are seen throughout the colon and evident from an early age; the risk of neoplasia is such that prophylactic colectomy is performed before the age of 20.

- Hereditary non-polyposis colon cancer (HNPCC): this is inherited in an autosomal dominant fashion and is due to mutations in DNA mismatch repair genes; individuals at risk are offered colonoscopic screening.

Epidemiology
The incidence of colorectal cancer increases with age, and overall has increased over the last 50 years. Colorectal cancer now accounts for 20,000 deaths per year in the UK.

Clinical presentation

Common

- Change in bowel habit: new-onset constipation or 'spurious' diarrhoea.

- Iron-deficiency anaemia.

- Rectal bleeding.

Uncommon

- Large bowel obstruction: constipation, pain and vomiting.

- Evidence of metastatic disease (ascites).

TABLE 40 FAMILY HISTORY AND LIFETIME RISK OF COLORECTAL CANCER. THERE IS A BENEFIT OF SURVEILLANCE COLONOSCOPY AT A RISK OF 1 IN 12 OR GREATER

Family history of colorectal cancer	Lifetime risk
None	1 in 40
One first-degree relative >45 years	1 in 17
One first-degree and one second-degree relative	1 in 12
One first-degree relative <45 years	1 in 10
Two first-degree relatives (any age)	1 in 6
Dominant inheritance (eg HNPCC)	1 in 2

HNPCC, hereditary non-polyposis colon cancer syndromes.

- Weight loss.

- Abdominal pain.

- Anorexia.

Physical signs

Common

In most cases there will be no diagnostic physical signs.

Uncommon

- Palpable abdominal mass.

- Signs of iron deficiency: pallor, koilonychia, glossitis.

- Signs of metastatic disease: hepatomegaly, ascites.

Investigation/staging

Dukes staging of colonic carcinoma (Fig. 54).

Blood tests

FBC, iron indices: may demonstrate iron-deficiency anaemia.

> Liver blood tests may be normal or there may be an isolated elevation in alkaline phosphatase (may be >1000 U/L) in the presence of liver metastases.

Tumour markers

Carcinoembryonic antigen (CEA) is not useful for diagnosis but may be useful in monitoring the patient's response to treatment and for the identification of disease relapse.

Colonoscopy

Colonoscopy is the investigation of choice. Total examination of the colon should be undertaken, even in instances of proven distal tumours, to exclude the presence of synchronous tumours or polyps. If this has not been performed prior to resection, it ought to be done subsequently.

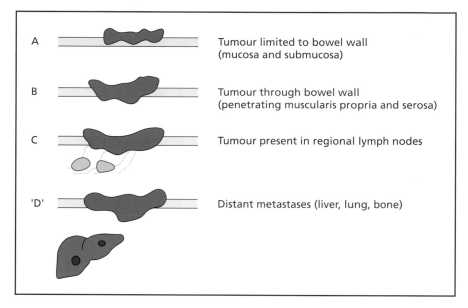

▲ **Fig. 54** Dukes staging for colorectal carcinoma. This was originally used for the staging of rectal cancer but is now widely adopted for colorectal cancer in general. Stage D was not originally described by Dukes.

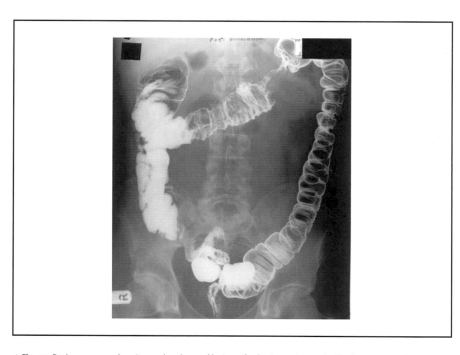

▲ **Fig. 55** Barium enema showing an 'apple-core' lesion of colonic carcinoma in the transverse colon.

Barium enema

May be considered in the elderly or frail, or where colonoscopy has been unsuccessful. Characteristic 'apple-core' lesions may be seen (Fig. 55).

Liver ultrasound, abdominal CT, MRI

Abdominal CT is now the investigation of choice for identifying metastatic disease. In patients with rectal carcinoma MRI scanning of the pelvis is used to determine invasion into local structures and determine suitability for resection. Chemotherapy or radiotherapy may be used prior to surgery in metastatic disease to down-grade the tumour stage, so staging should be performed except in emergency settings.

Differential diagnosis

Diagnoses listed in Table 41 should be considered.

Treatment

> It is not necessary to establish a tissue diagnosis before laparotomy if there are signs of impending bowel obstruction.

Emergency

Acute large intestinal obstruction is a surgical emergency with a high risk of caecal perforation.

Short-term

Surgery This is required in most cases of colorectal cancer. The extent of bowel resection depends on the site of the tumour: attempts are made to resect at least 5 cm of normal bowel either side of it.

Palliative approaches Although surgery is the usual treatment for patients with impending colonic obstruction, stenting of tumours with self-expanding metal stents offers an alternative approach for the palliative relief of obstruction.

Long-term or according to stage

Chemotherapy Treatment with 5-fluorouracil improves survival for Dukes' B and C cancers.

Radiotherapy Preoperative radiotherapy to 'down-stage' rectal tumours reduces local recurrence but has limited effect on survival.

Complications

Large bowel obstruction and metastatic disease are common.

Prognosis

Mortality

Prognosis following surgery depends on the histological grade of the

TABLE 41 DIFFERENTIAL DIAGNOSIS OF COLORECTAL CARCINOMA

Presentation	Diagnoses to consider
Change in bowel habit	Diverticular disease Irritable bowel syndrome Inflammatory bowel disease Gastroenteritis Thyroid disease
Iron-deficiency anaemia	Peptic ulcer disease Coeliac disease Upper gastrointestinal malignancy Colonic angiodysplasia Dietary deficiency (rare as sole cause)
Rectal bleeding	Haemorrhoids (fresh blood in the pan and on the paper) Diverticular disease (may cause massive bleeding; typically acute rather than persistent) Inflammatory bowel disease

TABLE 42 THE 5-YEAR SURVIVAL RATES AFTER RESECTION OF COLORECTAL CANCER

Dukes' stage	5-year survival (%)
A	95–100
B	65–75
C	30–40
Distant metastases	<1

tumour and the Dukes' stage (Fig. 54 and Table 42).

Prevention

Identifying asymptomatic individuals with premalignant or early malignant disease offers the opportunity to reduce the associated mortality of colorectal carcinoma. This is loosely referred to as 'screening', although it may be useful to distinguish 'targeted' screening on the basis of a pre-existing disease (surveillance, eg ulcerative colitis) or positive family history (case finding) from population screening of individuals of average risk.

Surveillance

Indications for surveillance include:

- previous diagnosis of colorectal cancer;

- previously identified colonic polyps (high-grade dysplasia, more than three adenomas, any polyp >1 cm);

- ulcerative colitis (initial surveillance colonoscopy at 10 years, then 3-yearly until 20 years, then 2-yearly until 30 years, then yearly);

- FAP syndrome;

- HNPCC or other familial colon cancer syndromes.

Case finding

Appropriate in those with a significant positive family history (see Table 40).

Population screening

Despite continuing controversy, population screening for colorectal cancer is shortly to be introduced in the UK. This will currently include all those over 60 years of age with a positive faecal occult blood test, and will eventually be extended to include those over 50 years old. Colonoscopy will be offered to all identified individuals at 5-yearly intervals.

> ⚠ Colonoscopy carries a risk of bleeding or perforation of 1 in 1,000, which is increased if therapeutic colonoscopy (eg polypectomy) is performed. Patients should be advised of this risk, including the potential need for surgery (perhaps colostomy) in such an eventuality.

FURTHER READING

Cairns S and Scholefield JH, eds. (Developed on behalf of the British Society of Gastroenterology and the Association of Coloproctology of Great Britain and Ireland). Guidelines for colorectal cancer screening in high risk groups. Gut 2002; 51 (Suppl. 5): v1–v2. Full text available at http://www.bsg.org.uk/

– – – – – – – – – – – – – – – – –

Weitz J, Koch M, Debus J, *et al*. Colorectal cancer. *Lancet* 2005; 365: 153–65.

2.9.3 Diverticular disease

Aetiology/pathophysiology/ pathology

Although there are suspicions that there may be an underlying genetic predisposition to diverticular disease, it is best considered as an acquired condition. Diverticula form as herniations of colonic mucosa through the muscularis layer. This process tends to occur more commonly in the distal colon and usually occurs at the point of entry of penetrating blood vessels through the muscle layers (hence the presentation with acute haemorrhage).

Epidemiology

The prevalence of diverticular disease of the colon increases with age: it is present in 50% of the population over the age of 50 years.

Clinical presentation

Common

Diverticula are common in elderly people, often asymptomatic and regarded as an incidental finding at colonoscopy/barium enema. Acute presentation is usually in the form of one of the common complications.

- Diverticulitis: an associated inflammation of the colon, often related to infection and thought to result from impaction of faeces within a diverticulum.

- Colonic bleeding: a frequent presentation of diverticular disease, thought to result from the fact that diverticula form at the point of maximal weakness in the colon, ie at the point where blood vessels penetrate the muscle coat.

Some patients will have non-specific symptoms such as low abdominal pain, constipation or diarrhoea.

Uncommon

- Diverticular abscess.

- Colovesical fistula.

- Colonic stricture: after repeated episodes of inflammation, resulting in subacute colonic obstruction.

Physical signs

There are no specific physical signs of diverticular change itself. In acute diverticulitis or in the presence of a diverticular abscess there may be left iliac fossa tenderness or a palpable mass.

Investigation

Barium enema/colonoscopy

Diverticular change may be demonstrated by either barium enema or colonoscopy.

Abdominal CT

CT is the best way to demonstrate abscess formation (Fig. 56). Colovesical fistulae require a high index of suspicion (recurrent urinary tract infections, pneumaturia, etc.) but may be identified on barium contrast radiology (Fig. 57).

Differential diagnosis

This includes colonic carcinoma, colonic ischaemia, inflammatory bowel disease and irritable bowel syndrome.

Treatment

Short-term

The management of diverticular disease is determined by the extent of symptoms or presence of complications. Acute diverticulitis requires intravenous fluids, antibiotics and analgesics, with diverticular abscess often requiring drainage in addition; bleeding will usually settle with supportive treatment.

Long-term

Avoidance of constipation (high-fibre diet, bulking laxatives such as Normacol, and good fluid intake) is recommended in the belief that this may reduce the risk of complications. Surgery is reserved for complicated diverticular disease (ie bleeding, abscess, stricture).

Prognosis

Many patients experience recurrent diverticulitis or bleeding, but diverticular change is not a progressive pathology and there is no increased risk of colonic neoplasia.

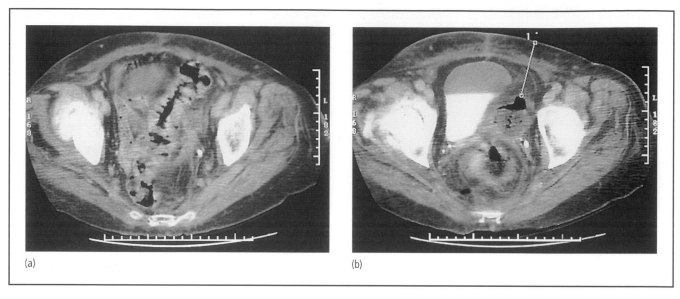

(a)   (b)

▲ **Fig. 56** Diverticular disease: (**a**) CT scan showing a loop of bowel (lumen in black) with diverticula; (**b**) adjacent collection (identified by tip of white marker line) due to a perforated diverticulum adjacent to the bladder.

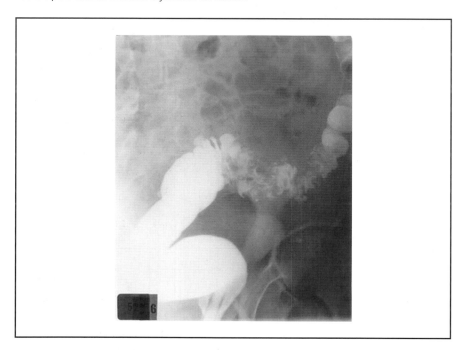

▲ **Fig. 57** Barium enema showing fistulae complicating diverticular disease.

FURTHER READING

Stollman N and Raskin JB. Diverticular disease of the colon. *Lancet* 2004; 363: 631–9.

2.9.4 Intestinal ischaemia

Aetiology/pathophysiology/pathology

As with vascular disease elsewhere in the body, the gut is prone to ischaemia from either progressive atheromatous narrowing of the mesenteric arteries or thromboembolism from intracardiac or proximal vascular sources.

Epidemiology

Vascular disease in general is increasing in most developed countries. Risk factors include age, male sex, family history, smoking, diabetes, hypertension, hyperlipidaemia and atrial fibrillation.

Clinical presentation

Common

Ischaemic colitis Bloody diarrhoea, usually of sudden onset and associated with abdominal pain.

> Ischaemia frequently affects the splenic flexure of the colon, which is the 'watershed' between areas supplied by the superior and inferior mesenteric arteries. The caecum and distal terminal ileum are also commonly involved.

Small bowel infarction This is usually due to arterial embolism and presents as an acute abdomen, often with severe systemic disturbance (hypotension, acidosis).

Uncommon

Mesenteric angina: recurrent postprandial abdominal pain and weight loss.

Physical signs

• Other features of atheroma: arcus, xanthelasma.

- Potential sources of arterial embolism: atrial fibrillation, heart valve disease.

- Abdominal bruits and other evidence of vascular disease.

Investigation

Radiological

- Plain abdominal radiograph: may show aortic calcification and colonic mucosal oedema, often with thumb-printing, which may be of relatively limited distribution compared with other forms of colitis (eg distal transverse colon and splenic flexure).

- CT or MRI angiography: the presence of significant stenosis or occlusion of two out of three (coeliac axis, superior mesenteric artery and inferior mesenteric artery) vessels is suggestive of significant disease; the superior mesenteric artery needs to be involved to justify intervention.

- Mesenteric angiography: confirms the radiological diagnosis and may allow therapeutic intervention to be performed (eg angioplasty or stenting).

Other

Colonoscopy may reveal ischaemic changes but carries increased risk of perforation in this context and is not recommended if ischaemic colitis is the most likely diagnosis.

Differential diagnosis

This includes colorectal carcinoma, diverticular change, inflammatory bowel disease, peptic ulcer disease and chronic pancreatitis.

Treatment

Acute intestinal infarction often requires emergency surgery for bowel resection. Lesser degrees of ischaemia (eg ischaemic colitis) are usually managed conservatively.

Complications

Intestinal strictures and obstruction.

Prognosis

Excess mortality is associated with other features of vascular disease (ischaemic heart disease, stroke, renal failure, etc.). Acute intestinal infarction carries a high mortality rate and significant long-term morbidity, often requiring parenteral nutrition.

FURTHER READING

Green BT and Tendler DA. Ischemic colitis: a clinical review. *South. Med. J.* 2005; 98: 217–22.

2.9.5 Anorectal diseases
See Table 43.

2.10 Liver disease

2.10.1 Acute viral hepatitis

2.10.1.1 Hepatitis A

Aetiology/pathology
Hepatitis A is an acute hepatitis caused by an RNA virus that is spread by the faecal–oral route. Figure 58 shows the histological picture of acute viral hepatitis.

Epidemiology
Hepatitis A is the commonest cause of viral hepatitis in the UK, with an incidence of symptomatic disease of about 6 per 100,000, most commonly between the ages of 20 and 45 years. Asymptomatic disease is common in childhood: 5% of children in the UK are immune by 5 years of age, compared with 74% of people over the age of 50 years.

Better sanitation means age of first exposure is increasing. Most cases are sporadic.

Hepatitis A endemic regions include, but are not limited to, Mexico, parts of the Caribbean, South America, Central America, Africa, Asia (except Japan), the Mediterranean basin, Eastern Europe and the Middle East. Hepatitis A remains the most common vaccine-preventable disease in travellers to endemic regions, who can contract hepatitis A by ingestion of contaminated drinking water or ice, uncooked fruits or vegetables grown with or washed in contaminated water, or raw or uncooked shellfish (oysters, clams or mussels). Outbreaks can be seen in day-care centres where children have not been toilet-trained, after breakdowns in usual sanitary conditions such as natural disasters, and occasionally through blood transfusions or by sharing contaminated needles and syringes. The incubation period is 15–45 days.

Clinical presentation

Common
Most cases are asymptomatic, with symptoms and severe disease more common with increasing age. If symptomatic the presentation is of an acute hepatitis with non-specific symptoms of lethargy, arthralgia, anorexia, nausea and mild upper quadrant discomfort (prodrome) followed by jaundice. The latter is associated with pale stools and dark urine. Itching can occur in the cholestatic phase of illness.

Physical signs
Features of an acute hepatitis (tender mild hepatomegaly, jaundice) are common. Splenomegaly is seen in 15% of cases.

TABLE 43 ANORECTAL DISEASES

Condition	Aetiology, pathophysiology, pathology	Clinical presentation	Investigation	Treatment
Haemorrhoids (piles)	'Varicose' perianal veins; associated with chronic constipation and straining at stool	Common findings are rectal bleeding (usually bright red blood on the toilet paper, but sometimes dramatic bleeding), perianal irritation (itching), pain (usually associated with thrombosis)	Proctoscopy Flexible sigmoidoscopy: necessary to exclude other causes of rectal bleeding (eg proctitis, rectal cancer, polyps) In some circumstances investigation of the more proximal colon by barium enema or colonoscopy may be necessary	Conservative: simple advice on diet, use of aperients and toilet habits Injection sclerotherapy (phenol) Banding: now replacing injection therapy Surgery: haemorrhoidectomy reserved for very troublesome haemorrhoids
Anal fissure	Tear in anal mucosa associated with straining and passage of a very hard constipated stool	Anal pain on defecation; constipation, which is sometimes secondary to the pain associated with defecation	Sigmoidoscopy and examination under anaesthetic	Conservative: advice on diet and hydration to avoid constipation GTN paste: when applied to the anus this leads to reduction in anal sphincter tone and healing of fissures Surgery: lateral sphincterotomy performed for resistant cases
Fistula in ano[1]	A fistulous tract originating in the rectum and opening onto the perineum or into other pelvic organs (most commonly the vagina)	Discharge: pus, mucus and blood may discharge spontaneously onto the perineum Pain: if persistent, usually indicates a complicating abscess	Sigmoidoscopy: but this may be very uncomfortable for the patient and may provide only limited information Examination under anaesthetic: allows thorough sigmoidoscopy and the probing of any identified tracts; biopsies should be taken to exclude Crohn's disease. MRI: is of increasing utility in delineating the course of fistulae and identifying associated abscess cavities	Conservative: advice on diet and hydration to avoid constipation Seton drain: a plastic drain placed through a fistula will keep the tract open and prevent the recurrent formation of abscess Fistulotomy: superficial fistulae may be laid open
Solitary rectal ulcer	Ulceration of the anterior rectal wall due to excessive straining. An increasing number of patients are presenting with rectal ulcers due to the use of nicorandil, a potassium channel agonist used in the treatment of ishaemic heart disease	Tenesmus and rectal bleeding	Sigmoidoscopy and rectal biopsy	Conservative: advice on diet and hydration to avoid constipation

1. Fistula in ano may cause faecal incontinence if it passes through the anal sphincter; Crohn's disease should always be considered in patients with recurrent or complex perianal fistulae.
GTN, glyceryl trinitrate.

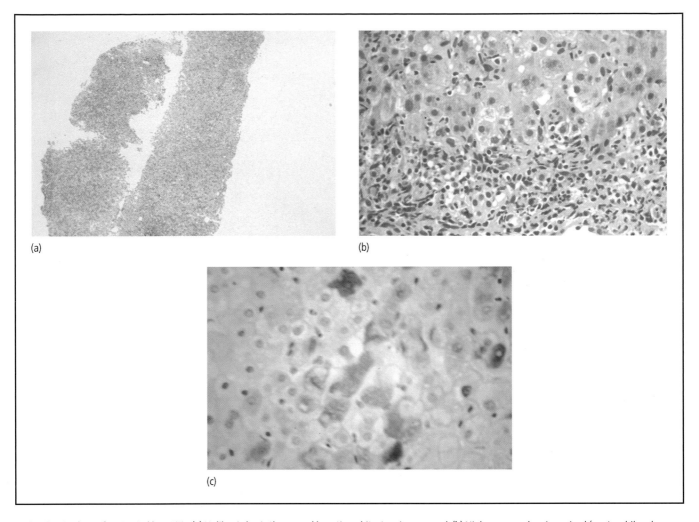

(a)

(b)

(c)

▲**Fig. 58** Histology of acute viral hepatitis. (**a**) Unlike cirrhosis the normal hepatic architecture is preserved. (**b**) Higher power showing mixed (neutrophil and polymorphonucleocyte) portal tract inflammation and infiltration of the lobule; other findings are hepatocyte necrosis and ballooning of hepatocytes. (**c**) Hepatitis B infection with positive immunohistochemical staining for HBsAg in hepatocytes.

Investigation

- Liver biochemistry: high serum transaminases (peak usually >1000 U/L), with or without raised serum bilirubin; alkaline phosphatase raised in cholestatic phase; normal albumin.

- Serology: the presence of hepatitis A IgM indicates a recent infection (Fig. 59).

Differential diagnosis

See Table 44.

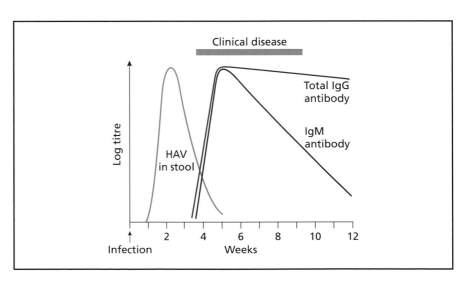

▲**Fig. 59** Serology in acute hepatitis A. HAV, hepatitis A virus.

TABLE 44 DIFFERENTIAL DIAGNOSIS OF ACUTE HEPATITIS

Common	Uncommon

Viral hepatitis
    Hepatitis A
    Hepatitis B (± hepatitis D)
    Hepatitis E
    Seronegative hepatitis
Drugs
    Paracetamol
    NSAIDs
    Flucloxacillin/Augmentin (co-amoxiclav)
    Dextropropoxyphene
Alcoholic hepatitis
Autoimmune chronic active hepatitis
Ischaemic hepatitis (eg heart failure, septic shock)
	Halothane
	Nitrofurantoin
	Liver infiltration (adenocarcinoma/lymphoma)
	Venous hepatic outflow obstruction
	Pregnancy-associated liver disease
	Wilson's disease

> In those with a typical hepatitis who are seronegative for hepatitis A and B, be sure to specifically request hepatitis E testing.

Treatment

This is supportive, with intravenous fluids if vomiting. Rare cases of acute liver failure need special management.

Complications

> A cholestatic phase in acute hepatitis is common, can last between 12 and 18 weeks, and is associated with rising bilirubin (ie 400–500 µmol/L) and alkaline phosphatase and falling serum transaminases. Relapsing disease is rare, occurring in 6%, but there is no chronic state.

Prognosis

Hepatitis A is self-limiting with no residual liver damage. Symptoms and signs usually resolve within 3 weeks. Acute liver failure occurs in 0.14–0.35%. Death occurs in 0.04% of patients with symptomatic disease.

Prevention

Passive immunisation

Pooled serum immunoglobulin can be given to close contacts of a case of hepatitis A within 2 weeks of exposure.

Active immunisation

Formalin-inactivated vaccine is indicated for travellers to high-risk areas, homosexuals, intravenous drug users and those with chronic liver disease. It provides protection for 5–10 years.

FURTHER READING

Kemmer NM and Miskovsky EP. Hepatitis A. *Infect. Dis. Clin. North Am.* 2000; 14: 605–15.

2.10.1.2 Other acute viral hepatitis

Hepatitis E

This is caused by hepatitis E virus (HEV), an RNA virus transmitted by the faecal–oral route. It accounts for sporadic and major epidemics of viral hepatitis, particularly in developing countries, but also in other parts of the world, eg 50% of non-A non-B (NANB) hepatitis in Hong Kong. It is rare in the UK, with only about 2% of adults being immune. There is low viral faecal excretion and hence low secondary spread.

Hepatitis E is seen in young adults and resembles hepatitis A. The incubation period is 34–46 days. Jaundice is often of sudden onset and liver biochemistry is cholestatic. Acute liver failure is rare. It is diagnosed by IgG and IgM antibodies to recombinant HEV proteins. Alternatively HEV RNA can be detected by polymerase chain reaction (PCR).

The disease is self-limiting. Acute haemorrhagic syndrome with encephalopathy and renal failure is a complication seen most typically in women in the last trimester of pregnancy and is associated with a 20% mortality.

Community-acquired hepatitis E infection does sporadically occur in the UK and should be considered as a cause of seronegative hepatitis. There is a suggestion that there may be an animal reservoir as the virus has been identified in a number of animal species including swine, sheep, cattle, poultry and rodents.

Cytomegalovirus

Cytomegalovirus (CMV) can cause an acute hepatitis, most commonly in those who are immunosuppressed. Patients may be asymptomatic, with hepatitis recognised solely from elevation of serum transaminases, but symptoms can range from fever and malaise to a devastating illness with jaundice and other features of CMV infection including pharyngitis, oesophagitis, gastroenteritis, pneumonitis, retinitis and bone marrow suppression. Diagnosis is by demonstrating CMV on tissue biopsy, detection of CMV by PCR in blood or urine, or by finding IgM to CMV. Treatment is with intravenous ganciclovir.

Epstein–Barr virus

Primary infection in children is asymptomatic. In young adults it can mimic viral hepatitis with fever and right upper quadrant pain together with elevated bilirubin (in 50%) and transaminases (up to 20 times normal). Diagnosis is made by a positive monospot or raised IgM to Epstein–Barr virus capsid antigens. The disease is self-limiting.

Other

Other rare causes of viral hepatitis include herpes simplex, adenovirus and rubella in the immunosuppressed. Parvovirus also rarely causes hepatitis in association with pancytopenia. Note that hepatitis C is not a cause of acute liver disease, but is the commonest cause of chronic hepatitis in the world.

FURTHER READING

Aggarwal R and Krawczynski K. Hepatitis E: an overview and recent advances in clinical and laboratory research. *J. Gastroenterol. Hepatol.* 2000; 15: 9–20.

2.10.2 Chronic viral hepatitis

Chronic viral hepatitis refers to inflammation of the liver (hepatitis) that is caused by a virus and which lasts for longer than 6 months. Hepatitis B and C viruses are the commonest causes. Presentation is highly varied: infection may be asymptomatic, subclinical causing only vague symptoms like fatigue, or lead to chronic liver disease and cirrhosis (about 20% of patients with chronic hepatitis B or C).

2.10.2.1 Hepatitis B

Aetiology/pathophysiology/ pathology

Hepatitis B virus (HBV) is a double-stranded DNA virus. The e antigen is a protein subunit of the core of the virus that is excreted by hepatocytes. Excess surface antigen is also found free in serum. The histological picture is of an acute hepatitis with liver damage due to immune clearance of the virus.

Epidemiology

Horizontal transmission is via parenteral transmission and sexual contact, and probably by close contact in young children. Vertical transmission accounts for the high rates of infection worldwide. The prevalence is falling, although worldwide there are still 350 million chronic carriers.

Clinical presentation

Common

Most infected individuals are asymptomatic. Some will have fever, malaise, nausea and right upper quadrant pain. Up to 4 months after exposure there may be self-limiting jaundice, which rarely lasts more than 1 month (Fig. 60).

Rare

A cholestatic phase and relapses are uncommon (unlike hepatitis A). The presence of immune complexes containing hepatitis B antigens leads to extrahepatic manifestations, eg polyarteritis, glomerulonephritis and myocarditis.

Physical signs

The acute phase may produce signs of an acute hepatitis. Signs of chronic liver disease develop later in some cases (see Section 1.2.2).

Investigation

Liver biochemistry

High serum transaminases and an elevated bilirubin may be seen in the acute phase.

Evidence of infection

Serological markers of HBV infection are shown in Table 45. During the acute phase of illness HBV DNA can be detected in the blood; this is cleared by 2 months in >90% of cases.

> Hepatitis B core IgM is often the only marker of infection in acute liver failure as the virus will have been eradicated by the immune system by the time liver failure occurs.

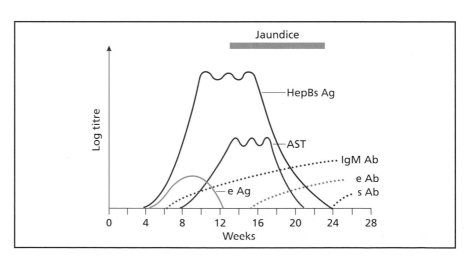

▲**Fig. 60** Time course of acute hepatitis B infection. AST, aspartate transaminases.

TABLE 45 SEROLOGICAL MARKERS OF HEPATITIS B INFECTION

	HBsAg	HBeAg	HBsAb	HBcAb (IgG)
Acute hepatitis B	+	+		
Resolved acute infection	–	–	+	+/–
Vaccination	+	–		

> Remember to tell a patient with HBsAg to avoid unprotected sexual intercourse unless his or her partner is immune to hepatitis B.

Treatment

No treatment is indicated for most patients with acute infection. Lamivudine is now being used in those with acute liver failure, and liver transplantation may be needed. In those with chronic active hepatitis, with evidence of ongoing inflammation biochemically and on liver biopsy, treatment with interferon alfa or lamivudine may be suggested after review by a specialist. Adevofir or entecavir may be used in the event of lamivudine resistance. Liver transplantation is offered for patients with decompensated hepatitis B cirrhosis.

Complications

Chronicity

Persistence of HBsAg in serum for longer than 6 months suggests chronicity. Overall, 10% of adults and 90% of neonates or those who become infected in infancy will become chronic carriers. The carrier rate in the UK is 0.1% compared with 10–15% in Africa. Chronicity is less common if the acute attack is more severe, ie associated with jaundice.

Acute liver failure

Due to enhanced immune response with rapid clearance of the virus.

Others

Polyarteritis and glomerulonephritis are rare.

Prognosis

Good unless acute liver failure ensues.

Prevention

Vaccination along with strategies to prevent exposure.

Children and adults

Recombinant vaccine is given intramuscularly; after three injections 94% will become immune. Low responders (often the elderly, the immunosuppressed or those on renal replacement therapy) may need a further booster/course of vaccination. For all receiving vaccination a booster is recommended every 5–7 years to maintain HBsAb levels above 100 IU/L. There is an argument for universal vaccination in childhood to eradicate HBV worldwide, but currently it is recommended for selected groups only (Table 46).

Neonates

If the mother has HBV, give hepatitis B immunoglobulin at birth as passive immunisation, together with hepatitis B vaccination.

2.10.2.2 Hepatitis C

Aetiology/pathophysiology/pathology

Hepatitis C virus (HCV) is an RNA virus that is parenterally transmitted, most commonly by percutaneous exposure to contaminated blood. Sexual transmission is possible, but not common. HCV infection occurs in 2–8% of infants born to HCV-infected mothers. Most of those infected develop hepatitis 14–160 days after exposure.

Epidemiology

In the UK, 0.1–0.5% of the population have been infected, but in some countries the prevalence is much higher, eg up to 20% in Egypt.

Clinical presentation

Most cases are asymptomatic: perhaps 20% develop a mild acute hepatitic illness, but jaundice is rare and symptoms are less severe than with hepatitis A or hepatitis B. In the long term, 85% of patients fail to clear the virus and have persistent viraemia. Many of these develop slowly progressive chronic liver disease, and over the course of 20–40 years progress from acute to chronic persistent hepatitis, to chronic active hepatitis, to cirrhosis (in 10%) and eventually hepatocellular carcinoma (1–4%).

TABLE 46 INDICATIONS FOR VACCINATION FOR HEPATITIS B

Surgical and dental staff[1]
Hospital staff in contact with blood products[1]
Mental abnormality
Close family and sexual contact of HBsAg-positive individual
Drug abusers
Homosexually active men
Travellers to high-risk areas

1. In many hospitals/healthcare settings, vaccination against hepatitis B is a condition of employment.

Physical signs

There are typically no abnormal physical signs in the acute stage of infection. Signs of chronic liver disease develop later in many cases (see Section 1.2.2).

Investigation

Liver biochemistry

In acute infection, alanine transaminase (ALT) typically rises to about 10 times normal and the bilirubin may also be increased. In patients with persistent HCV infection the ALT fluctuates indefinitely, but bilirubin returns to normal (until the development of advanced chronic liver disease).

Evidence of infection

HCV infection is usually diagnosed by testing for HCV antibodies. If positive this is followed by testing for HCV RNA, providing an independent method of confirming infection and determining whether it is persistent.

Liver biopsy

The acute hepatitis induced by HCV is generally less severe than with the other hepatitis viruses. In patients with persistent infection the histological findings can fluctuate, but scoring systems that typically quantitate necrosis, inflammation and fibrosis remain the best predictors of outcome and are often used to decide whether to offer antiviral treatment.

Treatment

Pegylated interferon alfa with ribavarin are effective but expensive and often difficult for patients to tolerate because of side effects. They should only be administered by specialists in accordance with recognised protocols.

Prognosis and complications

HCV infection is one of the commonest causes of chronic liver failure. Rare extrahepatic manifestations include membranoproliferative glomerulonephritis and mixed cryoglobulinaemic vasculitis.

Prevention

There is no vaccine for hepatitis C, hence prevention must be by reducing exposure.

FURTHER READING

Cramp M and Rosenberg W. *Guidance on the Treatment of Hepatitis C Incorporating the Use of Pegylated Interferons*. London, British Society for Gastroenterology, 2003. Full text available at http://www.bsg.org.uk/

- - - - - - - - - - - - - - - - - -

Ganem D, and Prince AM. Hepatitis B virus infection: natural history and clinical consequences. *N. Engl. J. Med.* 2004; 350: 1118–29.

- - - - - - - - - - - - - - - - - -

Poland GA and Jacobson RM. Clinical practice: prevention of hepatitis B with the hepatitis B vaccine. *N. Engl. J. Med.* 2004; 351: 2832–8.

- - - - - - - - - - - - - - - - - -

Poynard T, Yuen MF, Ratziu V and Lai CL. Viral hepatitis C. *Lancet* 2003; 362: 2095–100.

- - - - - - - - - - - - - - - - - -

Tan J and Lok AS. Update on viral hepatitis: 2006. *Curr. Opin. Gastroenterol.* 2007; 23: 263–7.

2.10.3 Acute liver failure

Aetiology/pathophysiology/pathology

Acute liver failure is distinguished from chronic liver disease by the absence of pre-existing clinical liver disease. Most simply, acute liver failure is defined as an acute illness of less than 26 weeks' duration, associated with coagulopathy (INR >1.5) and encephalopathy. Further classifications have been described.

- Hyperacute liver failure: encephalopathy occurring within 7 days of onset of jaundice, eg caused by paracetamol overdose.

- Acute liver failure: encephalopathy occurring within 8–28 days of jaundice.

- Subacute liver failure (previously known as late-onset hepatic failure): defined by encephalopathy that occurs between 5 and 12 weeks from onset of jaundice.

The conditions are characterised by acute hepatocellular necrosis. Causes are described in Section 1.4.6.

Clinical presentation

Increasing jaundice and confusion, ie encephalopathy, often following known precipitant, eg paracetamol overdose.

Physical signs

Jaundice and mild tender hepatomegaly. Small amounts of ascites may develop later. In hepatic venous outflow obstruction (Budd–Chiari syndrome) there is sudden onset of tender hepatomegaly and tense ascites.

Investigation and treatment

See Section 1.4.6.

> Patients should be discussed with or referred to a liver transplant centre sooner rather than later.

Complications

Common complications include the following.

- Cerebral oedema: occurs in 40–70% of patients who develop grade III/IV hepatic encephalopathy.

- Infection: bacterial in about 82% and fungal in 34% (often occult).

- Acidosis.

- Coagulopathy: but bleeding on account of coagulopathy is relatively rare.

- Renal failure: hepatorenal failure and/or acute tubular necrosis from paracetamol.

- Acute pancreatitis: seen particularly in paracetamol-induced toxicity.

Prognosis

Overall with medical treatment 10–40% of patients survive, with outcome best for paracetamol overdose and hepatitis A and worst for non-A non-B hepatitis and idiosyncratic drug reactions. The time to onset of encephalopathy is also a prognostic factor: 35% of patients with hyperacute failure survive compared with only 15% of those with subacute failure. With such figures, selection for transplantation is important and the 1-year survival after super-urgent liver transplantation probably now exceeds 65–75%.

Prevention

> Treatment of paracetamol overdose with *N*-acetylcysteine within 16 hours of overdose can prevent liver failure.

FURTHER READING

Khan SA, Shah N, Williams R and Jalan R. Acute liver failure: a review. *Clin. Liver Dis.* 2006; 10: 239–58.

2.10.4 Alcohol-related liver disease

In the UK, alcohol-related disease explains at least half of all clinical presentations of liver disease. It is estimated that 8% of men and 3% of women are 'problem drinkers', but many more people drink excessive amounts of alcohol (perhaps as many as 1 in 3 men and 1 in 5 women). About 20% of all adult inpatients admitted to general hospital settings are drinking in a hazardous or harmful way.

Aetiology/pathophysiology/pathology

Ethanol is primarily oxidised in the liver (Fig. 61). Men who drink more than 52 units or 420 g (1 unit of alcohol is 10 mL by volume, or 8 g by weight, of pure alcohol) per week and women who drink more than 35 units (280 g) per week are at increased risk of alcohol-related liver disease (ALD). The three most widely recognised forms of ALD are alcoholic fatty liver (steatosis), acute alcoholic hepatitis and alcoholic cirrhosis. The histology of alcoholic liver diseases is shown in Fig. 62.

Epidemiology

At least 80% of heavy drinkers develop steatosis, 10–35% develop alcoholic hepatitis and about 10% will develop cirrhosis.

Clinical presentation

Minor alcoholic hepatitis may be asymptomatic, with elevated serum transaminases as the only abnormality, and many people are diagnosed when they have routine liver function tests as part of a medical check-up. Severe alcoholic hepatitis presents with hepatic encephalopathy, jaundice, renal failure or coagulopathy. Other than those who present with decompensated liver disease, patients tend to have non-specific features such as nausea, vomiting, abdominal discomfort or diarrhoea. They may also present with other sequelae of alcoholism such as pneumonia, rib fractures, head injury, pancreatitis, neuropathy or heart failure.

Physical signs

This depends on the severity. Mild/moderate alcoholic hepatitis causes tender hepatomegaly, with jaundice in 10–15%. Severe alcoholic hepatitis causes jaundice, ascites, hepatic encephalopathy and rarely a hepatic bruit. Parotid gland enlargement and testicular atrophy are sometimes seen.

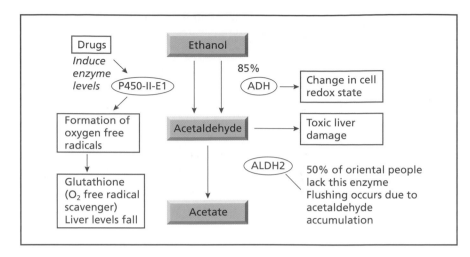

▲ **Fig. 61** Metabolic pathways involved in alcohol metabolism; 85% of alcohol is metabolised via the ADH pathway. ADH, alcohol dehydrogenase; ALDH2, acetaldehyde dehydrogenase 2; P450-II-E1, cytochrome P450-II-E1.

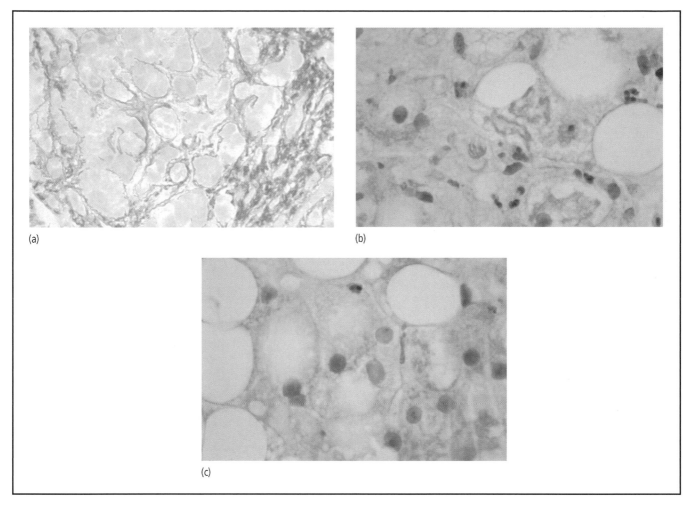

▲**Fig. 62** Acute alcoholic hepatitis. (**a**) Pericellular fibrosis around individual hepatocytes giving a 'chicken-wire' appearance. (**b**) Mallory's hyaline within hepatocytes. (**c**) Megamitochondria and fat within hepatocytes. Other features are predominantly neutrophil infiltration around portal tracts and fibrosis around the hepatic vein. More extensive fibrosis or established cirrhosis may also be present.

Investigation

Assessment of severity

- FBC: there is often a leucocytosis (more common with viral hepatitis) and a macrocytosis. An initial low platelet count is seen with acute alcohol use in the absence of portal hypertension. Low-grade haemolysis is common.

- Prothrombin time is an important prognostic marker.

- Liver function tests reveal aspartate transaminase (AST, usually >300 U/L) greater than alanine transaminase (ALT) in alcoholic liver disease. Alkaline phosphatase is often elevated, with levels up to three to four times normal in the absence of pancreatic disease (ie lower common bile duct stricture from chronic pancreatitis).

> Transaminase levels >1000 U/L are seen if there is associated paracetamol toxicity, which can occur with doses of as little as 4–6 g.

Assessment of chronic liver disease

Alcoholic hepatitis can coexist with other chronic liver diseases, eg haemochromatosis, hepatitis C and hepatitis B, which should be screened for as appropriate (see Sections 1.1.7 and 1.2.2).

Abdominal ultrasound is needed to exclude biliary obstruction and signs of portal hypertension suggestive of cirrhosis. Liver biopsy is diagnostic of acute alcoholic hepatitis but because of abnormalities in coagulation is not often performed in the acute context; in the long term it is needed to establish the extent of hepatic fibrosis.

Differential diagnosis

Drugs, viral hepatitis and autoimmune liver disease.

Treatment

This will depend on the presentation (see Sections 1.1.7, 1.2.2, 1.4.3 and 1.4.6) but with specific regard to alcoholic hepatitis and alcohol addiction.

Short-term

Corticosteroids should be considered in severe alcoholic hepatitis as long as there is no evidence of infection or renal failure.

Long-term

- Abstinence: psychological input and counselling both reduce readmission rates.

- Drugs: acamprosate and naltrexone (12 months) may reduce alcohol dependence. Disulfiram should probably be avoided because of side effects.

Complications

Ascites, hepatic encephalopathy, septicaemia, hepatorenal failure and chronic liver disease.

Prognosis

Patients admitted to hospital with alcoholic hepatitis have an overall 15% mortality at 30 days, but those with severe disease (hepatic encephalopathy, jaundice, renal failure or coagulopathy) have a mortality closer to 1 in 2. There are a number of ways of quantifying an individual patient's chance of surviving: the Maddrey discriminant function involves a formula including the prothrombin time and serum bilirubin, with those scoring highly (worse) often considered for a trial of steroids; the Glasgow Alcoholic Hepatitis Score (GAHS) depends on five variables (age, white blood cell count, urea, prothrombin ratio and serum bilirubin) and appears to perform slightly better. Overall survival at 5 years is 60% if the patient remains abstinent, falling to 40% if the patient continues to drink.

The development of complications of cirrhosis reduces life expectancy: a

first variceal bleed has an average in-hospital mortality of 20–30% and those with ascites have 50% mortality at 2 years. The treatment of hepatocellular carcinoma is usually palliative.

> Remember that although alcoholic liver disease has a poor prognosis, each patient should be assessed and managed on his or her own merits. Do not deny patients intensive care or organ support just because they are alcoholics.

Prevention

> Men should drink no more than 21 units of alcohol per week (and no more than 4 units in any one day) whereas women should drink no more than 14 units of alcohol per week (and no more than 3 units in any one day). Pregnant women who drink one or two drinks of alcohol (1 or 2 units), once or twice a week, are unlikely to harm their unborn baby, although the exact amount that is safe is not known.

Psychological input and counselling (including referral to Alcoholics Anonymous) is indicated when there is alcohol misuse.

Disease associations

These include hypertension, alcoholic cardiomyopathy, chronic pancreatitis, duodenal ulceration, peripheral sensory neuropathy, cerebellar atrophy, cerebral atrophy, Wernicke's encephalopathy and Korsakoff's dementia.

FURTHER READING

Bathgate AJ (on behalf of the UK Liver Transplant Units' Working Party). Recommendations for alcohol-related liver disease. *Lancet* 2006; 367: 2045–6.

Rueben A. Alcohol and the liver. *Curr. Opin. Gastroenterol.* 2007; 23: 283–91.

Sougioultzis S, Dalakas E, Hayes PC and Plevris JN. Alcoholic hepatitis: from pathogenesis to treatment. *Curr. Med. Res. Opin.* 2005; 21: 1337–46.

2.10.5 Drugs and the liver

2.10.5.1 Hepatic drug toxicity

Aetiology/pathophysiology/ pathology

Drug-induced liver injury is a potential complication of nearly every medication (prescribed or non-prescribed, pharmaceutical or herbal) since the liver is central to the metabolic disposition of virtually all drugs and foreign substances. Damage can occur to hepatocytes, bile ducts and hepatic veins, producing a range of clinical presentations (Table 47).

The effect of drugs on the liver may be predictable and dose dependent, eg paracetamol, but is more commonly idiosyncratic. Drugs can cause direct toxic damage, or indirect damage via the formation of reactive metabolites, which may deplete essential enzymes/cofactors, eg glutathione (paracetamol), or bind to liver proteins forming adducts. These adducts can subsequently mediate an immunoallergic response, eg autoantibodies to halothane and nitrofurantoin have been identified. Genetic factors are also important, eg deficiency in certain cytochrome P450 enzymes is associated with hepatotoxicity.

Histological features depend on the type of drug, but in general drug-induced liver damage may be differentiated from other causes of acute liver injury by the presence of large numbers of eosinophils (Fig. 63).

TABLE 47 CLINICAL PRESENTATIONS OF DRUG HEPATOXICITY

	Bilirubin	ALP/GGT	ALT/AST	Drug causes
Acute hepatitis	++	+	+++	Paracetamol
				NSAIDs
				Isoniazid
				Halothane
Acute cholestasis	+++	+++	+	Oestrogens
				Flucloxacillin
				Chlorpromazine
				Dextropropoxyphene
Fatty liver			++	Tetracycline
Steatohepatitis		++	++	Amiodarone
Granuloma	+	++		Carbamazepine
				Allopurinol
Hepatic fibrosis	N	N	N	Methotrexate
No liver disease (enzyme induction)		–/+		Rifampicin

ALP, alkaline phosphatase; ALT, alanine transaminase; AST, aspartate transaminase; GGT, γ-glutamyltransferase; N, normal liver biochemistry.

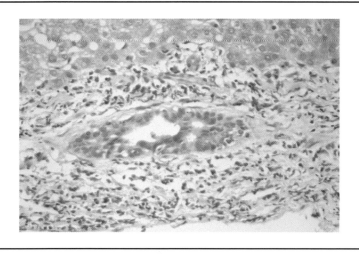

▲ **Fig. 63** Bile duct damage due to clavulinic acid–amoxicillin. The bile duct epithelium is irregular and infiltrated with lymphocytes.

Epidemiology

The incidence of hepatic drug toxicity is under-reported; it is thought to be 1 in 10,000–100,000. Prevalence increases with age, with drugs being responsible for 40% of acute hepatitis in those aged >50 years.

Drugs most commonly implicated in causing drug toxicity include:

- NSAIDs;
- paracetamol/dextropropoxyphene;
- clavulanic acid–amoxicillin (Augmentin);
- flucloxacillin;
- amiodarone;
- statins;
- thiopurines, eg azathioprine;
- HAART (highly active antiretroviral drugs);
- herbal remedies.

Clinical presentation/physical signs

⚠ Always consider drug toxicity in the presence of jaundice or abnormal liver biochemistry: always ask about over-the-counter and herbal remedies, and check with the patient's GP.

The clinical presentation depends on the type of liver injury.

- Jaundice: more likely if bile duct damage or cholestasis, but also occurs in severe hepatitis.

- Symptoms of hypersensitivity (fever, arthralgia) but these may be absent.

- Acute hepatitis: nausea and upper abdominal discomfort.

- Acute cholestasis: jaundice and itching.

- Fatty liver: usually asymptomatic.

⚠ There is usually a temporal association between starting a drug and the occurrence of hepatotoxicity, although liver biochemistry may become abnormal before symptoms develop. However, note that halothane and clavulanic acid–amoxicillin hepatotoxicity occur up to 3 weeks after cessation of drug exposure.

Investigations

FBC may show an eosinophilia. The pattern of liver biochemistry is shown in Table 47. Liver injury is defined as an ALT value more than three times the upper limit of the normal range, an ALP value more than twice the upper limit of normal, or a total bilirubin level more than twice the upper limit of normal if associated with any elevation of ALT or ALP. Liver injury is further classified as hepatocellular when there is a predominant initial elevation of ALT or as cholestatic when there is a predominant initial elevation of ALP; in a mixed pattern elevation of both values occurs.

Differential diagnosis

This depends on the type of liver injury caused by the drug.

- Acute hepatitis: viral hepatitis, autoimmune chronic active hepatitis, alcoholic hepatitis.
- Steatohepatitis: alcoholic hepatitis.
- Acute cholestasis: biliary disease, extrahepatic obstruction, intrahepatic disease (including primary sclerosing cholangitis, primary biliary cirrhosis and intrahepatic cholestasis of sepsis).

Treatment

Stop the drug. Supportive care. Ursodeoxycholic acid is often empirically prescribed for those with a cholestatic injury.

Complications

Acute liver failure

This is more likely in elderly people. It occurs in about 20% who are jaundiced. Overall 15–20% of acute liver failure is due to drugs. Frequently reported with antituberculous medication.

Chronic cholestasis

Loss of bile ducts (ductopenia) has been reported.

Prognosis

In the absence of liver failure most reactions are self-limiting with no chronic liver damage. If acute liver failure develops, outcome is not as good as that of viral hepatitis.

Disease associations

In severe reactions: erythroderma, bone marrow suppression.

2.10.5.2 Drugs and chronic liver disease

Clinical presentation

The following drugs should be avoided or used cautiously in patients known to have chronic liver disease.

- Narcotics/anxiolytics: accumulation results in hepatic encephalopathy.
- Codeine: causes constipation and secondary hepatic encephalopathy.
- NSAIDs: may cause haemorrhage from oesophageal varices and precipitate hepatorenal failure.
- Paracetamol: small overdoses can be fatal, hence caution should be exercised if the patient has decompensated liver disease.
- Gentamicin/radiocontrast agents: may precipitate hepatorenal failure.

Statins and liver disease

Postmarketing surveillance data suggest one case of liver failure for each million person-years of use, but there is no evidence of increased toxicity in those with pre-existing liver disease. Most guidelines recommend a baseline check of liver function tests before starting treatment, 8 weeks later and after any dose increase, then annual checks if tests are stable.

FURTHER READING

Arundel C and Lewis JH. Drug-induced liver disease in 2006. *Curr. Opin. Gastroenterol.* 2007; 23: 244–54.

Lee WM. Drug-induced hepatotoxicity. *N. Engl. J. Med.* 2003; 349: 474–85.

2.10.6 Chronic liver disease and cirrhosis

Aetiology/pathophysiology/pathology

Chronic liver disease is defined as liver damage persisting for more than 6 months. It results in progressive fibrosis and eventually cirrhosis (Fig. 64), which comprises fibrotic liver damage with regenerative nodule formation and consequent portal venous hypertension (Fig. 65).

Non-alcholic fatty liver disease can progress to cirrhosis, particularly when steatohepatitis is present and in those with diabetes and other metabolic syndrome features. Other common causes of chronic progressive liver disease are shown in Table 48.

Autoimmune hepatitis (relatively common) and Wilson's disease (very rare) can progress rapidly to cirrhosis, and indeed patients may be cirrhotic on presentation. Rapid progression to cirrhosis due to recurrent disease in the liver graft can also occur after liver transplantation, eg in recurrent hepatitis C or recidivist alcohol use. Rarer causes of chronic liver disease include sarcoidosis, biliary disease secondary to cystic fibrosis, long-standing biliary obstruction and chronic Budd–Chiari syndrome.

Epidemiology

Incidence varies with geographic region, age and sex. The commonest cause of chronic hepatitis in the world is hepatitis C; in the UK the commonest cause of cirrhosis is alcohol, followed by hepatitis C.

Clinical presentation

Common

- Non-specific malaise, loss of libido and mental changes.

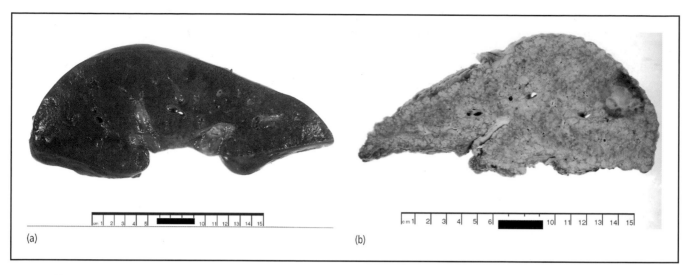

▲ **Fig. 64** (**a**) Normal liver; (**b**) cirrhotic liver containing a benign cyst.

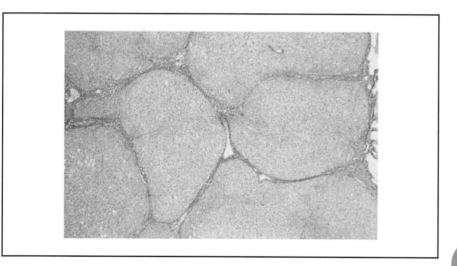

▲ **Fig. 65** Histological appearance of cirrhosis. There is loss of the normal architecture which is replaced by nodules.

- Hepatic decompensation: jaundice, ascites, hepatic encephalopathy, variceal haemorrhage.

> 🔑 Most patients with chronic liver disease are asymptomatic until they become cirrhotic, and cirrhosis may cause no symptoms until portal hypertension develops.

Physical signs
See Section 1.2.2.

Investigations/staging
See Sections 1.1.7 and 1.2.2 for discussion. Aside from the issues discussed in these scenarios, note that osteoporosis and more rarely osteomalacia are important complications of chronic liver disease and associated with significant morbidity through fractures resulting in pain, deformity and immobility. Patients with chronic liver disease should have their bone density measured, in addition to vitamin D and testosterone levels.

Treatment
See Sections 1.1.7, 1.2.2, 1.4.3 and 1.4.6 for discussion of the various clinical presentations that can arise in patients with chronic liver disease.

Specific measures
Progressive liver disease can sometimes be arrested where the cause is known (Table 49).

> ⚠️ **Wilson's disease**
>
> Wilson's disease may present as asymptomatic liver disease with predominant neurological abnormalities, as chronic liver disease with cholestatic features in early adulthood, or as fulminant liver failure in younger patients. A clue to Wilson's disease in these patients is the presence of significant red cell haemolysis. Always consider the diagnosis in patients under the age of 40 years with unexplained liver disease: prompt treatment can be life-saving.

General measures
Treatment is aimed at managing and preventing complications.

TABLE 48 IMPORTANT CAUSES OF CHRONIC LIVER DISEASE AND CIRRHOSIS

Alcohol-induced liver disease	See Section 2.10.4
Chronic viral hepatitis	Lobular lymphocytic infiltration, variable hepatocyte necrosis and fibrosis progresses to cirrhosis; damage is most likely due to immune-mediated mechanisms rather than a viral cytopathic effect
Genetic haemochromatosis	Excess iron absorption from the intestine results in accumulation in hepatocytes, hepatocyte necrosis and cirrhosis
Autoimmune liver disease	Immune cell infiltration and hepatocyte damage leads to rapidly progressing fibrosis and cirrhosis
Primary biliary cirrhosis	See Section 2.5.2
Primary sclerosing cholangitis	See Section 2.5.3
α_1-Antitrypsin deficiency	Abnormal protein cannot be adequately exported from hepatocytes, where it accumulates causing hepatocyte damage
Wilson's disease	Abnormalities in the biliary copper transporter results in excess copper accumulation in the liver and brain, with hepatocyte damage and basal ganglia disease The disease is genetically heterogeneous and this is reflected in variable clinical presentations (eg rapid neurological deterioration, early-onset fulminant liver failure, or chronic liver disease presenting with cirrhosis)

TABLE 49 SPECIFIC TREATMENT OPTIONS FOR VARIOUS CAUSES OF CHRONIC LIVER DISEASE

Cause of liver disease	Treatment
Alcohol-induced liver disease	Abstinence
Chronic viral hepatitis	Hepatitis C is cleared in more than 40% by a combination of interferon alfa and ribavirin (a nucleoside analogue) given for 6–12 months Hepatitis B responds to interferon alfa in 30% who are HBeAg positive with elevated transaminases. Antivirals including lamivudine, adevofir and entecavir are also used
Genetic haemochromatosis	Venesection to reduce iron load and return serum iron indices to normal reduces the rate of progression of liver disease (each venesection reduces ferritin by about 50 ng/mL)
Autoimmune liver disease	Systemic steroid treatment, with or without azathioprine, maintains long-term remission
α_1-Antitrypsin deficiency	No effective treatment exists
Wilson's disease	Penicillamine to increase urinary copper excretion and prevent hepatic and neurological disease progression Oral zinc may also promote copper excretion

HBeAg, hepatitis B e antigen.

- Ascites: diuretics, eg spironolactone, furosemide, amiloride.

- Portal hypertension: non-selective beta-blocker (propranolol).

- Bone disease: for osteoporosis/osteomalacia, treatments include calcium, bisphosphonates (eg cyclical etidronate, alendronate, risedronate), calcitonin and combined vitamin D/calcium.

- To maintain general health: nutrition.

> Refer patients with chronic liver disease for consideration of liver transplantation, particularly if complications develop or there is a deterioration in markers of liver function (albumin and prothrombin time).

Complications

Common

Coagulopathy Caused by decreased synthesis of coagulation factors II, V, VII and IX with worsening liver function, or as a result of chronic cholestasis and reduced levels of vitamin K. It is aggravated by thrombocytopenia caused by hypersplenism due to portal hypertension.

Encephalopathy The cause is multifactorial and ill-understood. Abnormal amino acid synthesis and increased ammonia production may play a role, as may abnormal enteric bacterial metabolism and reduced hepatic clearance of neurotoxic substances due to portal hypertension and shunting. Resting electroencephalogram shows slowed alpha-wave frequency. Treatments for encephalopathy are inadequate, but see Section 1.4.6 for discussion.

Ascites Results from a combination of portal hypertension, increased sodium and water retention, and hypoalbuminaemia. Spontaneous bacterial peritonitis (SBP) in cirrhotic patients with ascites is common and potentially fatal: prophylaxis with norfloxacin or ciprofloxacin should be considered. Regular paracentesis with human albumin infusions to maintain euvolaemia may be needed.

Hepatorenal failure Hepatorenal failure is a diagnosis of exclusion to be made only after the following causes of acute renal failure have been ruled out (which is often difficult to do): hypovolaemia (eg over-diuresis, bleeding), sepsis (particularly SBP), drug toxicity (eg NSAIDs, gentamicin, diuretics), intrinsic renal disease (eg IgA nephropathy) and urinary obstruction. The patient typically has a low urinary volume, with a low concentration of sodium in the urine, both persisting in the face of a fluid challenge. Treatment is supportive: some administer Glypressin with human albumin infusion to try to improve renal blood flow, but evidence of efficacy is weak. Prognosis is very poor.

Variceal haemorrhage The most common site is oesophageal and gastric varices, but varices can form at any site of contact between the portal and systemic circulation.

Cachexia As the liver is the primary regulator of glucose, lipid and protein metabolism, profound abnormalities occur with advanced liver disease and patients eventually become profoundly wasted. This is aggravated by haemorrhage, ascites, infection and anorexia.

Hepatocellular carcinoma Develops almost exclusively in cirrhotic livers, and patients with chronic viral hepatitis are most at risk, followed by those with haemochromatosis (Fig. 66). Hepatocellular carcinoma is less common in women of reproductive age. Development of hepatocellular carcinoma can precipitate ascites, encephalopathy and rapid hepatic failure.

Prognosis

Morbidity
There is significant morbidity from malaise, malnutrition, sepsis and bleeding. Figure 67 shows the natural history of hepatitis C infection.

Mortality
Life expectancy is severely reduced, but varies depending on the cause

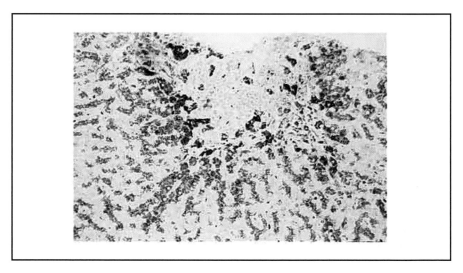

▲ **Fig. 66** Haemochromatosis: iron deposition in hepatocytes shown as blue staining with Perl's stain.

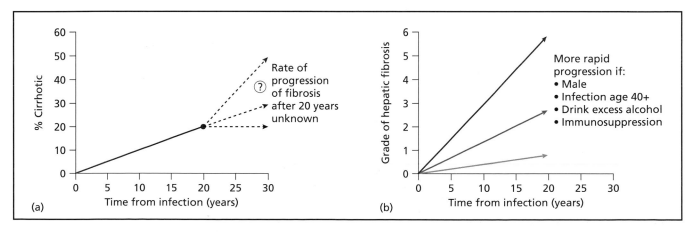

▲ **Fig. 67** Natural history of hepatitis C infection: **(a)** rate of progression to cirrhosis; **(b)** different rates of disease progression and factors associated with rapid progression.

123

TABLE 50 CHILDS–PUGH CLASSIFICATION

Parameter	Score		
	1	**2**	**3**
Bilirubin (μmol/L)[1]	<34	34–50	>50
Albumin (g/L)	>35	28–35	<28
PT (seconds prolonged)	<4	4–6	>6
Encephalopathy	None	Mild	Marked
Ascites	None	Mild	Marked

Childs–Pugh categories and their prognosis

	Total score	1-year survival
Class A	5–6	100%
Class B	7–9	80%
Class C	10–15	50%

1. If there is primary biliary cirrhosis or sclerosing cholangitis, then bilirubin is classified as 1 (<68 μmol/L), 2 (68–170 μmol/L) or 3 (>170 μmol/L).

and whether specific treatment is available (Table 49). Most patients die from sepsis, bleeding or progressive liver failure. Successful liver transplantation much improves the prognosis.

> There are many clinical scoring systems for liver disease, the simplest being the Childs–Pugh Classification (Table 50).

Iredale JP. Cirrhosis: new research provides a basis for rational and targeted treatments. *BMJ* 2003; 327: 143–7.

Moore KP and Aithal GP. Guidelines on the management of ascites in cirrhosis. *Gut* 2006; 55 (Suppl. 6): vi1–vi12. Full text available at http://www.bsg.org.uk/

FURTHER READING

Ginès P, Cardenas A, Arroyo V and Rodes J. Management of cirrhosis and ascites. *N. Engl. J. Med.* 2004; 350: 1646–54.

Ginès P, Guevara M, Arroyo V and Rodes J. Hepatorenal syndrome. *Lancet* 2003; 362: 1819–27.

Grant A, Neuberger J, Day C and Saxseena S (on behalf the British Society of Gastroenterology and the British Association for the Study of the Liver). *Guidelines on the Use of Liver Biopsy in Clinical Practice.* London: British Society for Gastroenterology, 2004. Full text available at http://www.bsg.org.uk/

2.10.7 Focal liver lesion

Aetiology/pathophysiology/pathology

The causes of focal liver lesions are shown in Table 51.

Clinical presentation

Common

- Abscess: fever, pain and tenderness.
- During investigation of abnormal liver tests.
- Incidental finding on ultrasound scanning.
- Detected on screening ultrasound in at-risk patients.
- Clinical deterioration or decompensation in cirrhotic patients.
- Onset of jaundice in patient with primary sclerosing cholangitis (PSC).

Uncommon/rare

Weight loss, abdominal pain, increased ascites secondary to portal vein thrombosis, and bleeding or tumour rupture.

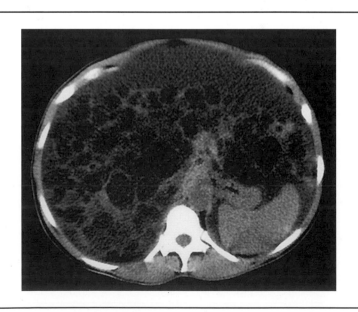

▲ **Fig. 68** CT scan showing multiple hepatic cysts in a patient with autosomal dominant polycystic kidney disease. The scan also shows ascites and absence of kidneys following bilateral nephrectomy.

TABLE 51 CAUSES OF FOCAL LESIONS IN THE LIVER

Type of cause	Condition	Comments
Infective	Pyogenic abscess Amoebic abscess Hydatid cyst	Often related to colonic disease or appendicitis Requires environmental exposure to *Entamoeba histolytica* Mainly in patients from agricultural regions; associated with exposure to dogs and sheep
Benign tumours	Simple cyst Haemangioma Hepatic adenoma Focal nodular hyperplasia/focal regenerative hyperplasia	Multiple cysts often found in adult polycystic kidney disease (Fig. 68) Extremely common, occurring in up to 20% of people, and detected usually as an incidental finding Occurs in 3–4 per 100,000 women on oestrogen-containing contraceptives, and may occur in men on androgen treatment
Secondary deposits	Colorectal cancer Other gastrointestinal tract cancer including pancreatic and carcinoid tumours (Fig. 69) Breast, cervix, ovary, prostate, lung, skin cancer	
Primary liver cancer	Hepatocellular carcinoma related to cirrhosis Cholangiocarcinoma Hepatocellular carcinoma developing in hepatic adenoma	Cell proliferation in regenerating cirrhotic nodules may favour malignant change, as may the effects of chronic viral infection on the host genome. Found in about 20–30% of patients dying with cirrhosis, particularly that caused by chronic viral hepatitis or haemochromatosis, and commoner in men than in premenopausal women Occurs in up to 15% of patients with primary sclerosing cholangitis Rare, except in inherited glycogen diseases

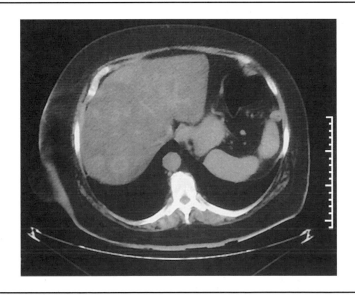

▲ **Fig. 69** CT scan showing multiple liver metastases from adenocarcinoma of the pancreas.

Physical signs

Common

There are often few signs but there may be:

- jaundice;

- signs of chronic liver disease in patients with hepatocellular carcinoma;

- hepatomegaly (tender in the case of liver abscess).

Uncommon

Hepatic bruit with hepatocellular carcinoma.

Investigations/staging

Blood tests

Any patient with a focal liver lesion will require routine blood tests including FBC, liver function tests, albumin, clotting screen and inflammatory markers. Some specific blood tests (Table 52) may help to confirm or refute a particular diagnostic possibility.

Imaging

Ultrasound scanning is most useful, but vascular tumours may have a diagnostic appearance on CT and MRI scanning and angiography, obviating the need for biopsy. Endoscopic retrograde cholangiopancreatography is useful for evaluating if jaundice in a patient with PSC is caused by

Test	Disease
Alpha-fetoprotein	Hepatocellular carcinoma; also acute hepatitis and germ cell tumours
CA19-9 tumour antigen	Cholangiocarcinoma; also other pancreatic and biliary diseases
Carcinoembryonic antigen	Colorectal carcinoma
Amoebic and hydatid serology	Past infection with amoeba or *Echinococcus* species

TABLE 52 BLOOD TESTS THAT CAN HELP TO ESTABLISH THE DIAGNOSIS OF A FOCAL LIVER LESION

cholangiocarcinoma, and allows collection of bile and brushings for cytological examination.

Tissue sampling

Histological diagnosis may be established by liver biopsy, but beware of vascular lesions that may bleed catastrophically on biopsy. If the patient has ascites, cytological examination may provide a diagnosis, particularly if the lesion is a secondary malignant deposit.

> ⚠ Beware of haemangiomas and hydatid cysts, where biopsy may result in catastrophic bleeding or disseminated infection.

Differential diagnosis

Common causes of focal liver lesions are shown in Table 51.

Treatment

Treatment of a focal liver lesion will depend on the cause. For benign lesions the most important aspect is to reassure patients that they have not got cancer.

Emergency

Liver abscess requires prompt antimicrobial treatment, and may require diagnostic or therapeutic aspiration or drainage. Rupture of liver abscess or haemangioma requires surgical intervention.

Short-term

Biliary obstruction can be relieved endoscopically or radiologically. Small hepatocellular carcinomas can be treated locally (eg by percutaneous alcohol injection, radiofrequency ablation, transarterial chemoembolisation), reducing tumour load and prolonging patient survival. Local resection of secondary deposits may be feasible in some cases.

Long-term

Pyogenic and amoebic liver abscess may be cured by antimicrobial treatment alone or combined with percutaneous drainage. Hydatid cysts usually require careful excisional surgery under antimicrobial cover.

Cessation of oral contraceptive use is associated with regression of adenomas. Benign neoplastic liver lesions may require surgical removal (partial hepatectomy or liver transplant) if there is a risk of major complications (usually impending rupture or haemorrhage). Early hepatocellular carcinoma may be cured by resection or liver transplantation.

Complications

Common

- Septicaemia in patients with pyogenic abscess.

- Decompensated liver failure in patients with cirrhosis or PSC.

Uncommon

Vascular thrombosis, particularly portal vein thrombosis or inferior vena cava thrombosis.

Rare

- Haemorrhage or rupture of haemangioma or large adenoma.

- Malignant transformation of adenoma.

Prognosis

Morbidity

Incidental liver lesions rarely cause morbidity. Fever, pain or vague right upper quadrant discomfort are common.

Mortality

Without curative resection hepatic secondaries and hepatocellular carcinoma usually have a dire prognosis.

> 🔑 **Hepatocellular carcinoma**
>
> Usually arises in the setting of cirrhosis, with untreated 1-year survival of 50–90% in patients with Childs–Pugh class A cirrhosis and 20% in those with Childs–Pugh class C disease. Metastases may develop in the lung, portal vein, periportal nodes, bones or brain, with 5-year survival rates less than 5% without treatment.
>
> Alpha-fetoprotein (AFP) is elevated in 75% of cases, and the higher the level the worse the prognosis. An elevation of greater than 400 ng/mL predicts hepatocellular carcinoma with specificity greater than 95%, and in the setting of a growing mass, cirrhosis and the absence of acute hepatitis, many centres use a level greater than 1000 ng/mL as presumptive evidence of hepatocellular carcinoma (without biopsy). However, two-thirds of hepatocellular carcinomas <4 cm have

AFP levels below 200 ng/mL, and up to 20% of hepatocellular carcinomas do not produce AFP even when very large. AFP values can fluctuate significantly in chronic hepatitis C and are therefore less useful for screening in this group of patients.

The only proven potentially curative therapy for hepatocellular carcinoma remains surgical, either hepatic resection or liver transplantation, and patients with a single small hepatocellular carcinoma (<5 cm) or up to three lesions <3 cm should be referred for assessment for these procedures. Hepatic resection should be considered as primary therapy in any patient with hepatocellular carcinoma and a non-cirrhotic liver (including fibrolamellar variant).

Screening by 6-monthly ultrasound and AFP measurement is generally advocated in those with cirrhosis, although there is no clear evidence of survival benefit.

Prevention

Primary

Low-dose oestrogen formulations reduce the risk of hepatic adenoma in patients using the oral contraceptive pill. The risk of hepatocellular carcinoma is reduced in patients with cirrhosis who abstain from alcohol and in patients with chronic viral hepatitis in whom viral replication is suppressed by antiviral therapies.

Disease associations

- Pyogenic liver abscess: cholangitis, diverticular disease, inflammatory bowel disease, appendicitis, colorectal neoplasia.
- Amoebic liver abscess: amoebic colitis.
- Adenoma: glycogen storage disease.
- Hepatocellular carcinoma: liver cirrhosis.
- Cholangiocarcinoma: PSC.

FURTHER READING

Choi BY and Nguyen MH. The diagnosis and management of benign hepatic tumors. *J. Clin. Gastroenterol.* 2005; 39: 401–12.

Garden OJ, Rees M, Poston GJ, *et al.* Guidelines for resection of colorectal cancer liver metastases. *Gut* 2006; 55 (Suppl. 3): iii1–iii8. Full text available at http://www.bsg.org.uk/

Llovet JM, Burroughs A and Bruix J. Hepatocellular carcinoma. *Lancet* 2003; 362: 1907–17.

Ryder SD (on behalf of the British Society of Gastroenterology). Guidelines for the diagnosis and treatment of hepatocellular carcinoma (HCC) in adults. *Gut* 2003; 52 (Suppl. 3): iii1–iii8. Full text available at http://www.bsg.org.uk/

2.10.8 Liver transplantation

Background

Over 600 adult orthotopic liver transplantations are carried out annually in the UK. Donor livers are matched to the recipient on the basis of size and ABO blood group. In contrast with renal transplantation, human leucocyte antigen (HLA) matching is not required. About 10% of those waiting will die on the list, which partly reflects a significant shortage of heart-beating brain-dead donors. Ways of trying to increase organ availability include the following.

- Living related transplantation: either a right or left lobe is used primarily in children who need small grafts, and in adults in Japan where cadaveric organs are not available because the concept of brain death is not recognised. This techinque is likely to be extended to adults in the UK in the near future.

- Split liver transplantation: this provides two grafts from a single donor and is useful in children. A minimum graft-to-donor weight ratio of 1% is needed to reduce the chances of so-called 'small for size' syndrome.

- Extending the use of marginal livers: most centres will now consider donation from patients of all ages, in those with evidence of past viral infection (hepatitis B and C), and in those with a history of certain malignancies.

- Non-heart-beating donors: the liver is sensitive to ischaemia, but criteria for controlled non-heart-beating donors (where death occurs in a hospital setting) are being developed and outcomes are good, although there is an increased risk of biliary complications.

- Xenotransplantation: this approach is not likely to be used in the near future despite all the research on using pig livers, mainly due to fears about transmissible infections.

Indications

Main indications for liver transplantation

- End-stage chronic liver disease.
- Acute hepatic failure.
- Metabolic liver disease: oxalosis, glycogen storage disease, hereditary amyloidosis.

Ethical issues

These are largely related to donor shortage and include the following.

- Should patients with liver failure due to paracetamol overdose or alcohol be transplanted?

- Should patients who have a worse post-transplant prognosis be transplanted (ie acute liver failure versus chronic liver disease)?
- Should patients with acute liver failure take priority over other patients already on a waiting list?
- Is there a role for xenotransplantation?

Emergency transplantation

There are two liver transplant waiting lists in the UK: acute liver failure (super-urgent list) and chronic liver disease. Strict criteria need to be met before an individual can be placed on the acute liver failure waiting list as these patients take priority over all other patients (Table 53).

Extent of liver dysfunction

The indication for liver transplantation in chronic liver disease is cirrhosis in the presence of hepatic decompensation, eg diuretic-resistant ascites, one episode of bacterial peritonitis, uncontrolled oesophageal variceal or gastric variceal bleeding, hepatic encephalopathy or a hepatocellular carcinoma <5 cm in diameter. Quality of life is also an important consideration. In the UK, patients are listed if they meet the indications for transplantation and are estimated to have >50% probability of survival after transplantation with a quality of life acceptable to the patient.

Timing of transplantation

Timing is a balance of risk of death without transplantation against risk with transplantation. Prognostic scores to assess mortality in chronic liver disease have been developed (eg Mayo score for primary biliary cirrhosis depending on albumin, prothrombin time and bilirubin) but are of limited value in individual patients. A decision as to when to list a patient for liver transplantation is also determined by the likely ease of organ procurement for that individual, this being more difficult if the patient is of small size or has blood group O or AB. Because of continued donor shortage it is likely that patients on the waiting lists will increasingly be prioritised on the basis of their probable mortality, ie the sickest patients will be transplanted first.

> ⚠ The waiting list for liver transplantation is up to 12 months, depending on the recipient blood group, and so early referral to a liver transplant centre is important. Patients with chronic liver disease do best if transplanted from home and most units will not transplant chronic patients from an intensive-care setting.

Contraindications

There are very few absolute contraindications to transplantation (eg cholangiocarcinoma, active bacterial infection) and patients should where possible be given the opportunity of assessment by a liver centre, but potential areas of concern include the following.

- Alcohol intake within the last 6 months: liver function can improve on abstinence, and this is also a risk factor for recidivism after transplantation. However, consideration should be given to patients who deteriorate before 6 months has elapsed if they are likely to remain abstinent.

- Increasing age, advanced end-stage disease, poor nutrition and cardiorespiratory disease.

- Psychiatric disease and absence of social support: may adversely affect compliance with immunosuppressive medication.

Note that HIV is not a contraindication to transplantation (if adequately treated).

Practical details

Surgery lasts between 4 and 24 hours and postoperative stays can be as short as 10 days, but are more typically 2–3 weeks. Anastomoses between donor and recipient hepatic artery, portal vein, inferior vena cava and biliary tree need to be fashioned and are sites of potential complications. Biliary anastomosis is usually a duct-to-duct anastomosis, but in the presence of recipient biliary disease (eg cystic fibrosis, primary sclerosing cholangitis) a Roux-en-Y biliary anastomosis is fashioned (Fig. 70).

Postoperative immunosuppression is typically with an initial combination of prednisolone and azathioprine/mycophenolate mofetil and

TABLE 53 KING'S COLLEGE HOSPITAL CRITERIA FOR LISTING FOR URGENT LIVER TRANSPLANTATION IN ACUTE LIVER FAILURE

Cause of acute liver failure	Criteria for listing
Paracetamol	pH < 7.3 or prothrombin time >100 seconds *plus* Creatinine >300 μmol/L *plus* Grade 3/4 encephalopathy
Non-paracetamol	Prothrombin time >100 seconds *or* any three of the following: Aetiology: drug reactions or non-A non-B hepatitis Age <10 or >40 Jaundice to encephalopathy in less than 7 days Prothrombin time >50 seconds Serum bilirubin >300 μmol/L

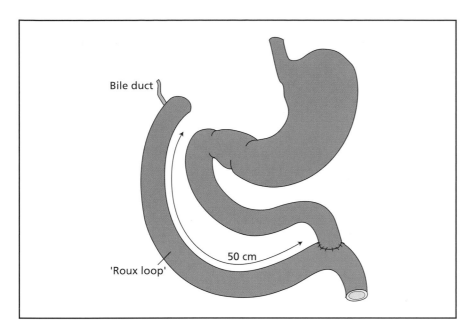

▲**Fig. 70** Roux-en-Y biliary anastomosis.

FURTHER READING

Clavein PA, Petrowsky H, DeOliveira ML and Graf R. Strategies for safer liver surgery and partial liver transplantation. *N. Engl. J. Med.* 2007; 356: 1545–59.

– – – – – – – – – – – – – – – –

Devlin J and O'Grady J (on behalf of the British Society of Gastroenterology). Indications for referral and assessment in adult liver transplantation: a clinical guideline. *Gut* 1999; 45 (Suppl. 6): vi1–vi22. Full text available at http://www.bsg.org.uk/

– – – – – – – – – – – – – – – –

Said A, Einstein M and Lucey MR. Liver transplantation: an update 2007. *Curr. Opin. Gastroenterol.* 2007; 23: 292–8.

tacrolimus, although many regimens now seek to avoid steroids completely. All patients require long-term immunosuppression, but this can often be with a single agent.

Outcome
The 1-year survival rate following transplantation for chronic liver disease is now approaching 95%, falling to 80% at 5 years primarily due to recurrent disease, cardiovascular events, malignancy and renal failure. The 1-year survival is only 61% following transplantation for acute liver failure, reflecting the presence of infection and multiorgan failure at the time of transplantation. Survival is lower following retransplantation, and in those receiving a liver and kidney at the same time.

Complications

Early complications
These include graft non-function and hepatic arterial or portal vein thrombosis, problems which usually require retransplantation. Up to 60%

of individuals have at least one episode of acute cellular rejection, usually occurring in the first few weeks, but unlike in renal transplantation this is not a predictor of chronic rejection, which only affects 5–10% of recipients.

Biliary complications
These affect 10–20% of patients and include anastomotic biliary strictures and biliary leaks.

Disease recurrence
The most important late complication is disease recurrence, including alcohol abuse; this may lead to graft loss before 5 years, particularly in hepatitis C and primary sclerosing cholangitis. Recurrent hepatic malignancy can be predicted by the proliferative index of the tumour on explant and the presence or absence of vascular invasion.

Comorbid illness
Malignancy, renal failure and cardiovascular events are increasingly being seen as recipients survive longer.

2.11 Nutrition

2.11.1 Defining nutrition

Nutritional requirements in health
A balanced diet supplies energy (fat and carbohydrate), nitrogen (protein), electrolytes and vitamins/trace elements. Fat is the most efficient storage form of energy, yielding approximately 10 kcal/g compared with glucose and protein (both 4 kcal/g).

Nutritional requirements vary depending on age, weight, degree of activity, growth, pregnancy and illness (catabolic states, eg sepsis, trauma, surgery). In health about 2,000–2,500 kcal of energy are required daily, as well as 14–20 g nitrogen (a minimum of 40–50 g protein). There are eight or nine essential amino acids (ie cannot be synthesised by humans) and one essential fatty acid (linoleic acid). Vitamins and trace elements are also required (Tables 54–56).

Assessment of nutritional status
The term 'malnutrition' includes both energy undernutrition and

TABLE 54 VITAMIN REQUIREMENTS (VITAMIN B IS COVERED SEPARATELY IN TABLE 55)

Vitamin	Requirement	Effect of deficiency	Notes
A	1000 IU/day	Night blindness, Bitot's spots, hyperkeratosis and keratomalacia of skin	Found in dairy products, liver, fish. Plasma retinol levels can be measured
C	60–100 mg/day	Scurvy	Necessary for collagen synthesis (hydroxylation of proline to hydroxyproline). Deficiency seen in the elderly or people who do not eat vegetables. Signs are perifollicular haemorrhages, 'corkscrew hair', bleeding gums, loose teeth, spontaneous bruising/haemorrhage, anaemia, poor wound healing. Vitamin C required to enable iron absorption
D	200 IU/day	Osteomalacia, rickets, bone pain, proximal myopathy, Looser's zones	Normal or low calcium, low phosphate, high ALP, high PTH. Main source is from action of sunlight on skin photoactivating 7-dehydrocholesterol. Dietary vitamin D hydroxylated in kidneys then liver to produce active compound
E	10–20 mg/day	Neurological disorders	Found in vegetable oils and fish
K	1 μg/kg daily	Bleeding diathesis	Found in leafy vegetables. Deficiency most commonly seen in biliary obstruction

ALP, alkaline phosphatase; PTH, parathyroid hormone.

TABLE 55 VITAMIN B REQUIREMENTS

Vitamin	Requirement	Effect of deficiency	Notes
B_1 (thiamine)	0.5–1 mg per 1000 kcal intake	Neuropathy, cardiac failure (beri-beri), ophthalmoplegia, (Wernicke's) encephalopathy, severe acidosis	Suspect in alcoholics, intravenous feeding with high glucose intake. Red cell transketolase levels can be measured
B_2 (riboflavin)	0.6 mg per 1000 kcal intake	Angular stomatitis, cheilosis, glossitis, conjunctival injection	Suspect in alcoholics. Can measure blood and urine levels
B_6 (pyridoxine)	1.6–2 mg/day or 0.038 mg/g protein intake	Angular stomatitis, cheilosis, glossitis, neuropathy, sideroblastic anaemia	Isoniazid, hydralazine and penicillamine are antagonists
Niacin	6.6 mg NE[1]	Pellagra (classically dermatitis 'Casal's necklace', diarrhoea, dementia)	Deficiency found in areas where maize is main dietary constituent (biologically unavailable niacin and low in precursor tryptophan)
Biotin	0.03–0.1 mg/day	Mental changes, myalgia, dermatitis	Deficiency rare
B_{12} (cobalamin)	2 μg/day	Megaloblastic anaemia, glossitis, stomatitis, peripheral neuropathy, subacute combined degeneration of the spinal cord	Found in meat, fish, dairy produce but not plants. Deficiency may occur in vegans, pernicious anaemia, gastrectomy, coeliac disease, bacterial overgrowth, ileal disease/resection, Zollinger–Ellison syndrome. Average adult stores may last up to 5 years before deficiency develops. Treat with 3-monthly vitamin B_{12} injections
Folic acid	3 μg/kg daily	Megaloblastic anaemia, glossitis, stomatitis	Found in green leafy vegetables and offal. Main cause of deficiency is poor intake. Deficiency may occur in small bowel disease (eg coeliac disease). Phenytoin and methotrexate are antifolate drugs

1. NE, niacin equivalent = niacin + tryptophan (mg)/60.

TABLE 56 MINERALS AND TRACE ELEMENTS REQUIRED IN DIET

Mineral	Requirement	Effect of deficiency	Notes
Iron	1 mg/day	Microcytic anaemia, glossitis, cheilosis, koilonychias	Iron deficiency is very common. Prevalence is 0.2% men, 1.9% postmenopausal women, 2.6% menstruating women. May be due to poor intake or excess loss (gastrointestinal tract most commonly)
Calcium	800–1000 mg/day is normal Western intake	Weakness, proximal myopathy, perioral paraesthesia, tetany	Correct for albumin level (add $0.02 \times [40 - \text{serum albumin}]$)
Copper	2–4 mg/day	Hypochromic anaemia, leucopenia, osteoporosis	
Magnesium		Myopathy	Deficiency common in alcoholics. Tends to follow calcium levels. Watch for associated hypokalaemia
Zinc	15 mg/day	Rash (nasolabial, hands), hair loss, infections, diarrhoea	
Selenium		Muscle pain and weakness, cardiomyopathy	
Chromium		Glucose intolerance, neuropathy	

overnutrition (eg obesity) as well as specific deficiencies or excesses of vitamins or trace elements. However, malnutrition is often used synonymously with undernutrition.

Nutritional assessment of patients in hospital is vital: almost half may be malnourished, and this is associated with increased mortality, higher incidence of hospital-acquired infections and prolonged hospital stay. There is no single adequate parameter of nutritional status. Assessment is mainly made by a combination of history and examination.

History

The following features from the history are important in assessing the nutritional state.

- Altered intake and pattern of intake.

- Recent weight loss (>10% significant).

- Ability to chew or swallow, presence of dysphagia.

- Anorexia, early satiety.

- Recent vomiting.

- Altered bowel habit suggesting malabsorption.

- Vitamin deficiency: angular stomatitis, glossitis, night blindness.

A number of screening tools have been used to identify patients at risk of malnutrition based on these features. Most have been shown to correlate poor nutritional status with adverse outcomes. Of these, the Malnutrition Universal Screening Tool (MUST, Fig. 71) is the easiest to calculate.

Examination

The following findings suggest impaired nutrition.

- General muscle and fat mass: hollow cheeks, wasting of temporalis, squaring of shoulders (loss of deltoid), wasting of quadriceps.

- Oedema: may indicate hypoalbuminaemia.

- Petechial or subcutaneous haemorrhage: consider vitamin C/K deficiencies.

- Wrinkling, dryness of conjunctiva: possible vitamin A deficiency.

- Ophthalmoplegia: thiamine deficiency; may be other signs of Wernicke's encephalopathy.

- Cheilosis, angular stomatitis, glossitis: vitamin B complex deficiency.

- Myelopathy, ataxia, retinopathy, blindness: vitamin E deficiency.

Body mass index

A nutritional assessment also involves calculating the body mass index (BMI) from the height (m) and weight (kg):

$$BMI = weight/(height)^2$$

The World Health Organization classifies BMI as follows:

<18.5	underweight
18.5–24.9	normal
25.0–30	overweight
>30	obese

Investigations

Blood tests Malnutrition may be indicated by albumin <30 g/L (but this usually reflects coexistent disease and is a very poor marker of nutritional state), lymphocytes

'Malnutrition Universal Screening Tool' ('MUST')

BAPEN
Advancing Clinical Nutrition

MAG
Malnutrition Advisory Group
A Standing Committee of BAPEN

BAPEN is registered charity number 1023927   www.bapen.org.uk

Step 1
BMI score

+

Step 2
Weight loss score

+

Step 3
Acute disease effect score

BMI kg/m²	Score
>20 (>30 Obese)	= 0
18.5–20	= 1
<18.5	= 2

Unplanned weight loss in past 3–6 months

%	Score
<5	= 0
5–10	= 1
>10	= 2

If patient is acutely ill and there has been or is likely to be no nutritional intake for >5 days
Score 2

If unable to obtain height and weight, see reverse for alternative measurements and use of subjective criteria

Step 4
Overall risk of malnutrition

Add Scores together to calculate overall risk of malnutrition
Score 0 Low Risk   Score 1 Medium Risk   Score 2 or more High Risk

Step 5
Management guidelines

0
Low Risk
Routine clinical care

- Repeat screening
  Hospital – weekly
  Care Homes – monthly
  Community – annually
  for special groups
  eg those >75 yrs

1
Medium Risk
Observe

- Document dietary intake for 3 days if subject in hospital or care home

- If improved or adequate intake – little clinical concern; if no improvement – clinical concern – follow local policy

- Repeat screening
  Hospital – weekly
  Care Home – at least monthly
  Community – at least every 2–3 months

2 or more
High Risk
Treat*

- Refer to dietitian, Nutritional Support Team or implement local policy
- Improve and increase overall nutritional intake
- Monitor and review care plan
  Hospital – weekly
  Care Home – monthly
  Community – monthly

* Unless detrimental or no benefit is expected from nutritional support eg imminent death.

All risk categories:
- Treat underlying condition and provide help and advice on food choices, eating and drinking when necessary.
- Record malnutrition risk category.
- Record need for special diets and follow local policy.

Obesity:
- Record presence of obesity. For those with underlying conditions, these are generally controlled before the treatment of obesity.

Re-assess subjects identified at risk as they move through care settings
See *The 'MUST' Explanatory Booklet* for further details and *The 'MUST' Report* for supporting evidence.

▲**Fig. 71** The Malnutrition Universal Screening Tool (MUST). (Reproduced with permission from BAPEN, and available from http://www.bapen.org.uk/.)

$<1.5 \times 10^9$/L or transferrin <2 g/L. Thyroxine-binding prealbumin and retinol-binding protein have been used as indicators of protein–energy malnutrition, but may be also affected by other conditions.

> ⚠ Although low albumin levels may indicate protein–energy malnutrition, albumin concentration often reflects disease activity and may be regarded as the 'reciprocal of the ESR' (erythrocyte sedimentation rate). Albumin has a plasma half-life of 21 days and although fasting affects albumin synthesis within 24 hours, this has little impact on albumin levels because of the low turnover rate and large pool size. Infection, malignancy, inflammation, and gastrointestinal, renal and liver disease may all depress albumin levels, and yet most anorexic patients have a normal serum albumin.

Anthropometric measurements
These include triceps and subscapular skinfold thickness, which provides an index of body fat, and the mid-arm circumference which provides a measure of muscle mass. However, there are problems with both the reference database and considerable interobserver measurement variability. Generally only used in trial settings.

Dynamometry This refers to the use of hand grip strength, which has been shown to predict postoperative complications in surgical patients. Other tests have used electrical stimulation of the adductor pollicis muscle in the hand to measure force–frequency curves, fatiguability and relaxation.

Others Delayed cutaneous hypersensitivity tests may also be used as indicators of nutritional status.

Total body water Body composition may be divided into four compartments: water, protein, fat and mineral. Total body water may be measured by isotope dilution techniques using tritium-, deuterium- or ^{18}O-labelled water. Water has a relatively stable relationship to fat-free body mass (protein), with the proportion of water taken to be a constant at 0.732. Hence measurement of total body water allows the following to be calculated:

Protein = fat-free body mass

Fat = [total body weight –
        (fat-free body mass + water)]

Combined non-invasive methods for measuring the following are in developmental stages:

- protein (total body nitrogen);
- fat (dual photon absorptiometry);
- mineral (dual photon absorptiometry and delayed γ neutron activation);
- water (isotope water dilution).

Prognosis
There is a near linear relationship of increasing BMI with morbidity and mortality. A BMI <15 kg/m^2 is also associated with increased mortality.

2.11.2 Protein–calorie malnutrition
Kwashiorkor and marasmus are the two classical primary nutrition disorders seen in children. Although described as distinct entities, features of both are often present. Marasmus is defined as present when weight is less than 60% that expected for the age, and is termed marasmic kwashiorkor when oedema is additionally present. Less severe protein–calorie malnutrition is present when weight is 60–80% that expected for age, and is termed undernutrition in the absence of oedema, and kwashiorkor in its presence.

Other causes of undernutrition include anorexia nervosa, intestinal disorders (eg Crohn's, coeliac), infections (including parasites), neoplasms and severe inflammatory disorders.

2.11.3 Obesity

> 🔑 'Sudden death is more common in those who are naturally fat than in the lean.' (Hippocrates)

Aetiology/pathophysiology
Obesity, defined as a BMI >30 kg/m^2, is a large and increasing problem. In addition to the total body-fat mass (estimated by BMI), the distribution of fat is also important. Truncal obesity is associated with dyslipidaemia, hypertension, insulin resistance, diabetes mellitus, cardiovascular disease and stroke. In clinical practice, the distribution of fat can be simply assessed by the waist/hip circumference ratio (WHR). The WHR should not exceed 1.0 in men and 0.85 in women. Genetic factors are involved. A signal protein, leptin, produced by adipose tissue, has recently been discovered that may modulate body weight and energy expenditure.

Epidemiology
In the UK, the prevalence of obesity increased from 8% in 1980 to 15% by 1995. In Europe and the USA the figures are 15–25%. As the BMI increases, so does morbidity and mortality. Obesity is a result of energy input exceeding output over a sustained period.

Treatment

Dietary
The principle of treatment is to induce negative energy balance,

which should be achieved by a combination of long-term low-intensity exercise and diet (500–600 kcal daily deficit), which should be low in fat. Some very low calorie diets may cause micronutrient deficiency, and should be monitored. Ketogenic diets such as the Atkins diet restrict the intake of carbohydrates and encourage eating fat and protein, which could have adverse long-term effects on health even if body weight is reduced.

Behaviour modification

Behaviour modification is important and includes a diary of food intake, meal frequency and separating eating from other activities. Regular exercise probably raises the basal metabolic rate and favours energy expenditure.

> Reducing energy intake by dietary modification and increasing energy expenditure by regular exercise are key to controlling obesity. Regular exercise probably acts partly by increasing the basal metabolic rate and favouring energy expenditure.

Drug treatments

These are considered if diet, exercise and behaviour modification has failed, and the risks of obesity outweigh the risks of the drug in that individual. Serotoninergic agonists suppress appetite but may cause pulmonary hypertension and pulmonary valve disease. Orlistat is a potent pancreatic lipase inhibitor that causes malabsorption of fats and has recently been shown to be effective in treating obesity, although a limiting side effect is that it produces a high incidence of steatorrhoea. Administration of appetite-suppressing hormones may provide an effective pharmacological treatment of obesity in the future.

Surgery

Vertical banded gastroplication, reducing the reservoir capacity of the stomach, is reserved for morbid obesity (BMI >35 kg/m^2). Jejunoileal bypass surgery is no longer performed because it causes severe hepatic abnormalities.

Other issues

Other cardiovascular risk factors present in the obese patient should be addressed (eg smoking, hypertension, diabetes, hyperlipidaemia), and alcohol intake should be minimised (7 kcal/g). Hypothyroidism should be excluded.

FURTHER READING

Dietz WH and Robinson TN. Clinical practice: overweight children and adolescents. *N. Engl. J. Med.* 2005; 352: 2100–9.

Farooqi S and O'Rahilly S. Genetics of obesity in humans. *Endocr. Rev.* 2006; 27: 710–18.

Li Z, Maglione M, Tu W, *et al.* Meta-analysis: pharmacologic treatment of obesity. *Ann. Intern. Med.* 2005; 142: 532–46.

McNatt SS, Longhi JJ, Goldman CD and McFadden DW. Surgery for obesity: a review of the current state of the art and future directions. *J. Gastrointest. Surg.* 2007; 11: 377–97.

2.11.4 Enteral and parenteral nutrition and special diets

Principle

Nutritional support is indicated for malnourished patients and those at risk of malnutrition, for example through debilitation, surgery, reduced consciousness or disease of the gastrointestinal tract. Support may be given enterally (gastrointestinal) or parenterally (intravenous).

Indications

Enteral nutrition

Enteral nutrition is the preferred option in all malnourished patients who have a normal or near-normal, functioning, accessible gut. It is trophic for the upper intestinal mucosa, maintains epithelial barrier integrity, and is cheaper and safer than parenteral feeding. If the upper gastrointestinal tract is obstructed, for example by oesophageal disease, a percutaneous enterogastrostomy (PEG) tube can be used to bypass the obstruction and maintain enteral feeding.

Parenteral nutrition

Parenteral nutrition is indicated in those malnourished patients who have a non-functioning gut (eg short bowel syndrome, prolonged ileus). Traditionally, parenteral nutrition is administered via the large central veins (subclavian or internal jugular), which allows rapid dilution of the hyperosmolar solutions and reduces the incidence of thrombophlebitis and subsequent line failure. The introduction of lipid suspensions allowed total nutritional supplementation intravenously in a realistic infusion volume over a realistic time-frame, ie total parenteral nutrition (TPN).

Contraindications

Enteral nutrition

This is contraindicated in paralytic ileus, mechanical obstruction and major intra-abdominal sepsis, and in those with complex fluid balance problems.

Practical details

Enteral nutrition

Many patients can take oral supplements (eg Fortisip, Fortijuice) by mouth. In those with swallowing problems or those who lack appetite, nasogastric feeding may be initiated via a fine-bore feeding tube. A PEG or percutaneous enterojejunostomy (PEJ) tube may be sited if long-term enteral feeding is required, as these are more convenient and comfortable than a nasogastric tube and not prone to removal/ displacement. Nasojejunal feeding may be the preferred option in patients in whom aspiration is a potential problem, eg gastric dysmotility.

Parenteral nutrition

Venous access is secured via the internal jugular, subclavian or antecubital veins. A tunnelled central venous catheter should be sited unless it is anticipated that feeding is only required for a few days.

Complications

Parenteral nutrition

The complications of parenteral nutrition include central venous access-related complications, metabolic complications, vitamin and trace element deficiencies and hepatobiliary dysfunction. The metabolic complications include hyperglycaemia/hypoglycaemia, hypernatraemia/hyponatraemia, hypercalcaemia/hypocalcaemia and magnesaemia, hypophosphataemia, mineral/vitamin/trace element deficiency and cholestatic jaundice.

> Enteral nutrition is always preferred to parenteral nutrition: even small volumes of enteral feeding can help to maintain intestinal health and hasten the ultimate return to normal feeding.

Special diets

Elemental diet

This comprises low-molecular-weight nutrients, usually with 10% free amino acids, 85% oligosaccharides and <5% fat. It is as effective as steroids in the treatment of active Crohn's disease, but many patients find it distasteful and need nasogastric feeding over a 6-week period. Its mechanism of action is unknown, but it may exert its effect by reducing immunogenic load and altering bacterial flora.

Exclusion diets

The most common conditions requiring exclusion of specific foods from the diet are coeliac disease (where gluten provokes an immunological response), cows' milk protein intolerance and hypolactasia. Some patients with irritable bowel syndrome seem to benefit from avoiding certain foods.

Diets for weight loss

Restricting calorie intake reduces body weight, although homeostatic mechanisms probably act to counteract changes in the long term, frequently resulting in rebound weight gain after a few months. Some diets restrict fluid intake, with dehydration causing rapid but spurious weight loss. To maintain weight control, diets must be sustainable, nutritionally adequate, and not lack essential vitamins, minerals or macronutrients. Very low calorie diets carry the risk of undernutrition and should be supervised by a physician, while low-calorie diets such as those advocated by Weight Watchers are safer. The Atkins diet advocates avoidance of carbohydrates and favours a relatively high intake of fats and proteins, with the lack of carbohydrate promoting ketogenesis from fats and the high protein content possibly suppressing appetite and resulting in loss of weight. Long-term consequences may include dyslipidaemia, vitamin and mineral deficiencies, and possibly an increased risk of colorectal cancer, which is associated with a diet rich in meat products and deficient in insoluble fibre.

FURTHER READING

Baldwin C, Parsons T and Logan S. Dietary advice for illness-related malnutrition in adults. *Cochrane Database Syst Rev 2007; (1): CD002008.*

Milne AC, Potter J and Avenell A. Protein and energy supplementation in elderly people at risk from malnutrition. *Cochrane Database Syst Rev 2005; (2): CD003288.*

National Collaborating Centre for Acute Care. *Nutrition Support for Adults: Oral Nutrition Support, Enteral Tube Feeding and Parenteral Nutrition. Methods, Evidence and Guidance.* NICE guideline CG32. London: National Institute for Health and Clinical Excellence, 2006. Full text available at http://www.nice.org.uk/

Stroud M, Duncan H and Nightingale J. Guidelines for enteral feeding in adult hospital patients. *Gut 2003; 52 (Suppl. 7): vii1–vii12.* Full text available at http://www.bsg.org.uk/

Zaloga GP. Parenteral nutrition in adult inpatients with functioning gastrointestinal tracts: assessment of outcomes. *Lancet 2006; 367: 1101–11.*

3.1 General investigations

The main function of the gastrointestinal tract is to absorb nutrients, hence disease of the intestine frequently manifests with nutritional deficiency. Loss of weight, which can be assessed by estimating BMI, is a useful general test. Low body mass may arise from general debilitation, cachexia due to malignancy, malabsorption caused by intestinal or pancreaticobiliary disease, chronic liver disease, or chronic inflammatory disease such as Crohn's or ulcerative colitis.

Anaemia and nutritional deficiency

> The FBC is an extremely useful general test in gastroenterology: anaemia may be caused via many mechanisms that involve the gastrointestinal tract.

Deficiency of a number of key nutrients can manifest as anaemia. Iron deficiency is the most common nutritional defect worldwide. It may be due to inadequate intake, malabsorptive disease such as coeliac disease, occult gastrointestinal bleeding due to peptic ulceration, colorectal cancer or blood loss due to intestinal helminth infestation. Furthermore, chronic inflammation, including inflammatory bowel disease, can result in relative malabsorption of iron and anaemia.

Anaemia may also be caused by deficiency of vitamin B_{12} or folic acid. Deficiency of vitamin B_{12} may reflect disease of the stomach (post gastrectomy, atrophic gastritis) or terminal ileum (post resection, or due to ileal Crohn's disease), and is very rarely due to inadequate intake (eg in vegans). Folic acid is found mainly in green leafy vegetables and predominantly absorbed in the jejunum. Deficiency may be dietary or caused by chronic infestation and inflammation of the jejunum, eg giardiasis.

Serum biochemical tests

> In gastroenterological practice hypoalbuminaemia may reflect nutritional disease, liver disease or inflammatory disease.

Hypoalbuminaemia may be a sign of severe nutritional deficiency, be part of the acute-phase response to systemic inflammation or may be due to severe liver dysfunction. The serum alkaline phosphatase level may be raised due to disease of the intestine. Acute-phase proteins such as C-reactive protein are sensitive markers of inflammation that can reflect the activity of conditions such as Crohn's disease.

Stool examination

Determining relevant facts about the amount and composition of stool is a key aspect of the gastroenterological assessment. Stool may also be examined for occult blood, fat globules, leucocytes, erythrocytes and pathogens. Normal stool volume is about 200 mL per day, and the normal frequency of defecation varies from approximately three times a day to once every 3 days. Examples of abnormalities in the stool and their interpretation are shown in Table 57.

TABLE 57 ABNORMALITIES OF THE STOOL

Abnormality	Interpretation
Volume >200 mL/day	Diarrhoea: may indicate secretory diarhoea if this persists during an enforced fast
Fat globules visible (steatorrhoea)	Fat malabsorption: pancreatic or biliary disease is likely
Fecal occult blood test positive	Ingestion of raw meat products, excessive red meat consumption, occult intestinal bleeding
Leucocytes present	Intestinal inflammation or dysentery
Pathogenic bacteria, ova or cysts of parasitic species	Intestinal infection or infestation

3.2 Tests of gastrointestinal and liver function

The main measure of gastrointestinal function is determined by clinical history-taking. Most blood tests, radiological investigations and endoscopic modalities do not give a measure of function but quantify structural abnormalities and damage. However, there are a number of tests used to determine whether there has been disruption of normal physiology, which will be considered in anatomical order.

Oesophageal manometry and pH monitoring

Gastro-oesophageal reflux and associated pathology (especially Barrett's oesophagus and oesophageal adenocarcinoma) are assuming greater public health importance. Measuring gastro-oesophageal motility and acid reflux are important adjuncts to endoscopy and radiology and can be performed simply in an outpatient setting. A nasogastric tube is passed and pH or pressure measurements taken through an appropriate transducer and recording apparatus. The results are used to determine whether oesophageal symptoms (heartburn, pain, dysphagia or odynophagia) are related to acid reflux or abnormal oesophageal motility and whether surgical intervention may be useful.

Pancreatic function tests

Direct tests

Secretin–caerulein test Duodenal intubation test where pancreatic juice enzyme concentration and bicarbonate are analysed following injection of secretin. This test is considered the gold standard but is invasive, time-consuming and not routinely performed in many UK centres.

Lundh test meal A duodenal intubation test similar to the secretin–caerulein test but the stimulus is a specially formulated test meal. Similarly invasive to the secretin–caerulein test but gives information about gut signalling to the pancreas.

Indirect tests

Faecal fat Either by Sudan staining of stool sample or microscopy. This has gone out of favour as it involves the patient consuming a large volume of fat in the diet for 3 days after stopping any pancreatic supplements. It is insensitive in mild to moderate pancreatic insufficiency as greater than 90% of acinar tissue needs to be lost before the test becomes abnormal.

PABA test/mixed triglyceride breath test/pancreolauryl test/triolein breath test A complex substrate is administered orally, which is hydrolysed by the pancreatic enzymes and then absorbed by gut, with products measured in blood, urine or breath.

Faecal enzyme measurement Pancreatic chymotrypsin and elastase have both been developed into commercial tests, although faecal elastase appears to be superior. Enzymes are released from the pancreas, pass through the intestine without degradation and can be measured in a single stool sample. Low levels are associated with reduced exocrine pancreatic function.

Small bowel function

Measuring small bowel function is challenging and many methods are currently still research tools. Two types of test are most commonly employed.

Stool tests: collecting samples over a period of days and measuring weights and volume can help to determine the difference between osmotic diarrhoea and secretory diarrhoea. This can be enhanced by fasting the patient.

Breath tests: bacterial metabolism or intestinal absorption of orally administered substrates forms the basis of a number of functional tests. In some cases the products of metabolism result in the release of H_2 or CO_2 gas, which is detected on the breath; alternatively, renal excretion of substrate is measured. Some commonly performed tests are described in Table 58.

Other tests of small bowel function include gut permeability tests, using chromium-labelled EDTA administered orally. Motility disorders can be investigated using small bowel manometry, when a long catheter with pressure transducers along its length is passed fluoroscopically or endoscopically and then left to take measurements throughout a determined time period. The migrating motor complex (MMC) is propagated in the stomach and passes down the small intestine with gathering intensity, with different periods of activity such as the interdigestive period and nocturnal patterns. Pressure measurements can be used to characterise different types of pseudo-obstruction and other clinical applications are being developed, but it is not in routine use in many centres.

Liver function tests and liver damage tests

The conventional liver function tests do not reflect liver function: bilirubin, the transaminases and alkaline phosphatase give information on liver damage more than function. The most sensitive and specific

TABLE 58 FUNCTIONAL AND BREATH TESTS USED IN GASTROENTEROLOGY

Investigation	Indications	Substrate	Metabolite/read-out	Notes
Urease breath test	*Helicobacter pylori* infection	^{13}C-labelled urea	^{13}C-labelled CO_2	Most sensitive and specific test for *H. pylori* infection
Lactose breath test	Hypolactasia	Lactose	Excess H_2 from bacterial fermentation of lactose	
Lactulose breath test	Intestinal bacterial overgrowth and intestinal hurry	Lactulose	Early release of excess H_2 by bacteria in the small intestine, or as a result of rapid intestinal transit	Lactulose is not absorbed or metabolised by the intestine and normally reaches the large intestine intact
Glycocholate breath test	Intestinal bacterial overgrowth	Labelled glycine-glycocholate	Early release of labelled glycine by bacteria in the small intestine results in absorption of glycine and release of labelled CO_2 in the breath	
Xylose excretion test	Malabsorption due to small intestinal disease	Xylose	Urinary xylose excretion	Most ingested xylose is normally excreted unchanged by the kidneys, unless it is not absorbed
Schilling test	Cause of vitamin B_{12} deficiency	Labelled hydroxocobalamin (vitamin B_{12}) tracer administered after body stores are saturated by an intramuscular dose of unlabelled vitamin B_{12}	Urinary excretion of labelled vitamin B_{12}	Normal: complete absorption and excretion of vitamin B_{12}. Pernicious anaemia: incomplete absorption and excretion of vitamin B_{12}, corrected by co-administration of intrinsic factor Terminal ileal disease: incomplete absorption and excretion of vitamin B_{12}, not corrected by co-administration of intrinsic factor

measure of liver function is the prothrombin time (PT), which is simple to measure and reproducible. Other tests of liver function include the plasma urea (the urea cycle predominantly occurs in the liver), serum glucose concentration (gluconeogenesis) and serum albumin, but all are also affected by factors other than liver function. Urea is affected substantially by renal function and protein intake, glucose can be altered by comorbid conditions, and albumin falls in many acute severe illnesses as the liver switches to production of acute-phase proteins.

3.3 Diagnostic and therapeutic endoscopy

Endoscopy of the intestinal tract is one of the most powerful diagnostic and therapeutic manoeuvres available to the physician and can be safely performed under light sedation even in frail and ill patients. Originally flexible fibreoptic devices with a light source and a channel for suction, insufflation and instrumentation were used, but these are now increasingly replaced by devices

that collect visual information through a charge-coupled device located at the end of the instrument. Channels for insufflation, suction and instrumentation are still present, but the visual information is transmitted electronically and viewed on a video-display unit. The main endoscopic procedures are shown in Table 59 (apart from endoscopic retrograde cholangiopancreatography: see Table 61).

TABLE 59 ENDOSCOPIC TECHNIQUES FOR EXAMINING THE INTESTINAL LUMEN

Investigation	Indications/abnormalities	Contraindications/notes
Oesophago-gastroduodenoscopy (upper gastrointestinal endoscopy)	Causes of dyspepsia, including peptic ulcer Causes of heartburn, including gastro-oesophageal reflux disease Causes of haematemesis, melaena and iron-deficiency anaemia	Ensure that endoscopy is safe (eg that the patient's airway is protected, and the patient understands the procedure) A frail patient with cardiac failure or respiratory compromise should not be endoscoped without due attention to these problems Dysphagia may be caused by carcinoma of the oesophagus, which could be perforated on endoscopy: consider a barium or gastrograffin swallow first Endoscopy may be therapeutic as well as diagnostic, particularly in the treatment of upper gastrointestinal haemorrhage, including adrenaline injection, thermal or mechanical treatment of bleeding ulcers, or the banding of oesophageal varices. May also enable dilatation of benign strictures or the stenting of obstructing tumours. Biopsy obtained for urease assay (CLO test) can diagnose *H. pylori* infection at the bedside. Patients should preferably abstain from acid-suppressing medications for 2 weeks prior to the test Duodenal biopsy should always be performed when investigating iron-deficiency anaemia to exclude coeliac disease
Enteroscopy	A special long endoscope may be introduced beyond the duodenum, but the technique is unreliable	There is no reproducible and reliable endoscopic means of examining the small intestine between the second part of the duodenum and the terminal ileum. The advent of wireless capsule endoscopy has altered the potential to visualise the small bowel. Predominantly of use in the investigation of iron deficiency and/or recurrent gastrointestinal haemorrhage that defies other diagnostic techniques. May enable targeted endoscopic therapy by enteroscopy or surgery. May occasionally diagnose small bowel diseases such as Crohn's disease. Should be avoided in patients with obstructive symptoms
Colonoscopy and terminal ileoscopy	Colitis, colorectal polyps, carcinoma, diverticulosis Terminal ileitis, ileal Crohn's disease and tuberculosis Mucosal lesions such as angiodysplasia that are not detected radiologically	Requires adequate colonic clearance (eg with polyethylene glycol-containing purgative) There is a risk of colonic perforation and bleeding of ~1 per 1,000 cases, particularly if laser treatment, electrocautery or polypectomy is performed May be diagnostic (eg altered bowel habit, iron deficiency) or therapeutic (eg polypectomy, colonic stenting of obstructing tumours)
Flexible sigmoidoscopy	Colonic lesions distal to the splenic flexure	Does not require extensive colonic purging: may be performed after an enema. May be useful as a screening test, or to assess the extent of ulcerative colitis

CLO, *Campylobacter*-like organism.

3.4 Diagnostic and therapeutic radiology

Choosing the best imaging modality can be difficult. If in doubt, discuss with a radiologist.

Luminal radiology

The lumen of the intestine can be imaged by introduction of radio-opaque contrast or air (Table 60). Although still images are usually studied, much of the information comes from dynamic changes, so consultation with the radiologist supervising the procedure is essential to obtain maximal diagnostic information (Fig. 72).

Pancreaticobiliary investigations

The main pancreaticobiliary investigations are summarised in Table 61.

Radiological investigations for occult blood loss and iron-deficiency anaemia

Upper gastrointestinal endoscopy (oesophago-gastroduodenoscopy) and colonoscopy will provide a

TABLE 60 RADIOLOGICAL INVESTIGATION OF THE GASTROINTESTINAL LUMEN

Investigation	Indications/abnormalities	Contraindications/notes
Barium or Gastrograffin swallow	Oesophageal dysmotility, stricture, neoplasia, rupture or fistula	Barium should be avoided if there is high suspicion of rupture, fistula or potential for aspiration, when Gastrograffin (water-soluble contrast) is preferred Barium swallow should precede endoscopy when investigating dysphagia
Barium meal	Stomach and duodenal ulcers, gastric outlet obstruction, surgical anastomoses	Endoscopy is the preferred modality to investigate most gastric and duodenal pathology, but barium meal may be useful particularly in the postsurgical stomach
Barium meal and follow-through or small bowel enema	Diseases of the small intestine: lymphoma, tumours, Crohn's disease, Meckel's diverticulum	Relatively insensitive and non-specific; dependent on expert interpretation
Barium enema	Colorectal carcinoma, polyps, diverticulosis, complications of IBD	Contraindicated in frail or immobile patients who are unable to position themselves on the radiology table and who may be overcome by the strong purgative necessary beforehand Contraindicated for 24 hours after rectal or colonic biopsy Alternative to colonoscopy that does not allow therapeutic manoeuvres such as polypectomy or collection of tissue for histology
Defecating proctogram	Assessment of obstructive defecation	Useful in planning whether surgical intervention may be needed
Endoanal ultrasound	Assessment of faecal incontinence	Identification of sphincter damage
Transabdominal ultrasound	May demonstrate thickening of the intestinal wall in IBD Location and characterisation of intra-abdominal collections	User dependent May be used to direct drainage of collections or target biopsy of masses
Contrast CT scanning and virtual colonoscopy	Colorectal carcinoma, polyps, diverticulosis, complications of IBD	Used interchangeably with barium enema Air insufflation of the colon is well tolerated and allows delineation of the lumen Abnormalities of the wall can be detected Imaging is improving rapidly as image-processing software evolves
MRI scanning	Assessment of Crohn's disease	Particularly useful for identifying fistulous tracks in the perineum

IBD, inflammatory bowel disease.

diagnosis in most cases of gastrointestinal bleeding, but may need to be repeated if the bleeding is intermittent or due to a small, easily missed lesion. Other techniques may also be used, particularly for blood loss from the small intestine, which is inaccessible to endoscopy (Table 62).

3.5 Rigid sigmoidoscopy and rectal biopsy

The rectum and distal sigmoid colon can be viewed directly with a rigid instrument and a light source. Many symptomatic colorectal carcinomas occur distally, and patients with ulcerative colitis almost universally have rectal involvement.

Indications

- Altered bowel habit.

- Rectal bleeding of unknown cause.

- Diarrhoea and rectal bleeding in patients with ulcerative colitis.

- Tenesmus, proctalgia.

- To obtain rectal mucosal biopsy, eg for diagnosis of schistosomiasis, amyloidosis.

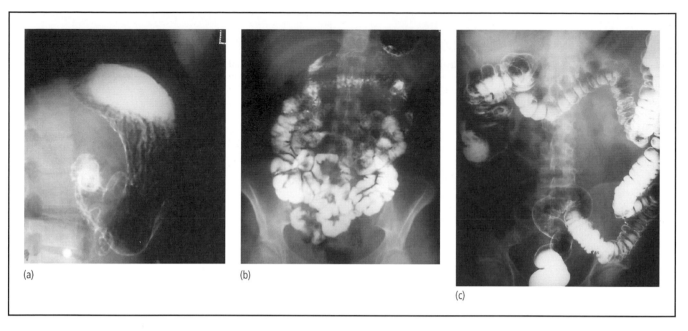

▲ **Fig. 72** Normal barium studies: (**a**) barium meal; (**b**) barium follow-through; and (**c**) barium enema.

TABLE 61 PANCREATICOBILIARY INVESTIGATIONS

Investigation	Indications/abnormalities	Contraindications/notes
Ultrasound scan	Dilated intrahepatic ducts Dilated extrahepatic ducts Stones Gallbladder wall abnormalities Pancreatic abnormalities	Initial investigation of choice for suspected biliary and pancreatic disease, although pancreas often obscured by overlying bowel (Fig. 73). Fasting avoids postprandial gallbladder emptying and increases sensitivity CT and MRI scanning may add further information, especially with intravenous contrast agents
Endoscopic retrograde cholangiopancreatography (ERCP)	Dilated or strictured bile ducts Typical features of PSC ('beads on a string' stricturing) Carcinoma of the head of the pancreas Stones	Contraindications as for any upper gastrointestinal endoscopy Side-viewing endoscope allows cannulation of the ampulla of Vater, with radiocontrast injection demonstrating biliary tree on fluoroscopy Allows sampling/brushing/biopsy May be therapeutic, eg retrieval of stones, sphincterotomy, insertion of stent
CT scanning	Cancer staging Further delineation of pancreatic abnormalities	Gives more detailed information than ultrasound especially in pancreatic disease Can be used to direct biopsy
Percutaneous transhepatic cholangiography (PTC)	Dilated or strictured ducts	Caution if there is disordered coagulation or low platelet count Radiocontrast is introduced into the biliary system by percutaneous injection Indicated when ERCP is difficult or impossible May be therapeutic as well as diagnostic, eg allows cutaneous drainage of bile from an obstructed system and stent insertion
Magnetic resonance cholangiopancreatography (MRCP) (see Fig. 24)	Intrahepatic and extrahepatic biliary and pancreatic anatomy Can also detect solid parenchymal lesions and thickening of bile ducts	Cannot be performed in some patients with metallic implants and electrical devices Claustrophobia is a relative contraindication Increasingly used as it is non-invasive and does not use X-rays Imaging is improving as software and machines evolve
Functional testing	HIDA (radionuclide) scanning Bromsulphthalein excretion test	HIDA scanning demonstrates functional biliary excretion and is useful for delineating complicated surgical anastomoses, biliary leaks, etc. Bromsulphthalein excretion is a measure of biliary excretory function

PSC, primary sclerosing cholangitis.

TABLE 62 INVESTIGATION OF OCCULT GASTROINTESTINAL BLOOD LOSS

Investigation	Details/indications/abnormalities	Notes
Red cell scanning	Patient's red cells are radiolabelled and reinjected. A gamma camera is used to locate the site of radioactive accumulation, which corresponds to extravasation of blood	Requires relatively brisk bleeding, eg 100 mL per 24 hours May not provide sufficient anatomical detail to direct therapy
Meckel's scanning	Technetium label directed to parietal cells	Detects ectopic gastric mucosa, which may be associated with a Meckel's diverticulum
Selective visceral angiography	Brisk bleeding from the coeliac or mesenteric arterial territories	Requires fairly brisk bleeding to be detected, eg 750 mL/day May be therapeutic (embolisation of vascular lesion)
Exploratory laparotomy	Reserved for young patients where an anatomical lesion such as Meckel's diverticulum is more likely	Often inadequate to locate subtle mucosal abnormalities such as angiodysplasia May be combined with 'on table' endoscopy, especially for the small intestine

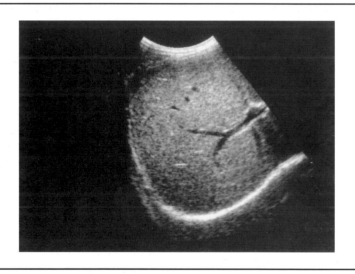

▲ **Fig. 73** Normal ultrasound of the liver. The liver has normal texture and the bile ducts are not dilated.

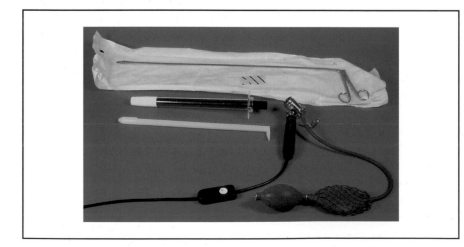

▲ **Fig. 74** Disposable plastic sigmoidoscope with obturator removed, light source and insufflator with rubber bulb, and sterilised packaged 'crocodile' biopsy forceps.

Contraindications

Sigmoidoscopy cannot be performed if:

- the patient is unwilling, apprehensive or uncooperative;

- there are inadequate facilities (lack of privacy, nurse escort or chaperone, biopsy forceps);

- severe anorectal pain (consider examination under anaesthetic);

- biopsy contraindicated in presence of bleeding diathesis.

Practical details

Before the procedure

The procedure can usually be performed without an enema beforehand. Ensure that the patient's clotting and platelet count are satisfactory. Sedation or intravenous cannula are unnecessary.

Essential equipment (Fig. 74) includes a sigmoidoscope with obturator, light source, insufflating bulb with functioning ball valve, and biopsy forceps. Lubricating jelly, swabs, towels, gloves and a specimen pot with histological fixative should be at hand.

Ensure that the patient understands the procedure, and that a nurse or assistant is present to reassure the patient, hand you additional equipment and act as a chaperone.

The procedure
Explain the procedure and place the patient comfortably in the left lateral position, with the buttocks close to the edge of the couch and the knees slightly extended. Perform a gentle rectal digital examination. Lubricate the sigmoidoscope and obturator. With the obturator fully inserted in the sigmoidoscope, insert the first 5 cm of the instrument into the anus, pointing anteriorly and cranially (towards the umbilicus). Withdraw the obturator and attach the light-source head and insufflator. Gently insufflate air and direct the instrument posteriorly (towards the sacroiliac joint) until a luminal view is obtained. Insert the instrument gently, insufflating and manoeuvring to maintain a luminal view. Examine the mucosa in all directions by angling the instrument gently. The instrument may safely be inserted to 20 cm provided a mucosal view is maintained and the patient does not complain of discomfort. If indicated obtain a mucosal biopsy by inserting a forceps through the viewing port, and gently shearing a sample of mucosa under direct vision. Withdraw the instrument to 5 cm, carefully examining the mucosa. Replace the obturator and remove the instrument.

It is safest to take a biopsy posteriorly and from the distal 10 cm where the rectum lies outside the peritoneum. The procedure should be painless provided the anal mucosa is avoided.

After the procedure
Warn the patient that there may be minor rectal bleeding for about 24 hours if a biopsy has been taken. Complications are rare, but may include pain, bleeding and perforation.

3.6 Paracentesis

Paracentesis can be diagnostic or therapeutic. A diagnostic paracentesis involves the removal of 50 mL ascitic fluid using a sterile green needle and syringe. The fluid should be analysed for albumin, amylase, cytology and a quantitative white count. Inoculate blood culture bottles with ascites to increase the chance of growing pathogens. If the fluid is cloudy, then chylous ascites is confirmed by an ascitic triglyceride level greater than the serum level.

Indications

All patients with ascites must have a diagnostic ascitic tap.

Therapeutic paracentesis is used as treatment of tense diuretic-resistant ascites in patients with portal hypertension.

Contraindications
Absolute contraindications are small or large bowel obstruction with dilated loops of bowel, and clinically evident fibrinolysis/disseminated intravascular coagulation. Most physicians routinely correct coagulation if the INR is >2 and/or transfuse platelets if the platelet count is $<50 \times 10^9$/L, but there is no evidence that this is required if the patient has no clinical evidence of bleeding.

Practical details

Before the procedure
Lie the patient flat on the back. Prepare the following equipment: suprapubic bladder drainage catheter or paracentesis catheter (Fig. 75), lidocaine 1 or 2%, blade, suture, urine catheter bag, 10-mL syringe and 18G needle.

The procedure
Insert the catheter into either the right or left iliac fossa. Clean the skin and infiltrate with lidocaine through to the peritoneum: do not continue with the procedure if you are unable to draw back ascitic fluid while anaesthetising. Make an incision in the skin. Insert the catheter through the skin and angle it obliquely for 1 cm or so before entering the peritoneum at 90° to the skin and a little way from the skin entry site. This reduces the risk of an ascitic leak on removal of the catheter. Secure the catheter with adhesive dressings: most liver units remove paracentesis catheters after about 6 hours so a suture is not usually indicated. Attach the end of the catheter to the urine bag. Tape the catheter securely to the abdominal wall.

Allow 5–10 L of ascites to drain over 1–6 hours: if the fluid does not drain, change the patient's position. In patients with portal hypertension give 6 g albumin intravenously per litre of fluid drained (100 mL 4.5% albumin = 4.5 g; 100 mL 20% albumin = 20 g).

After the procedure

Remove catheter after 6 hours irrespective of the amount of fluid drained to reduce the risk of bacterial peritonitis.

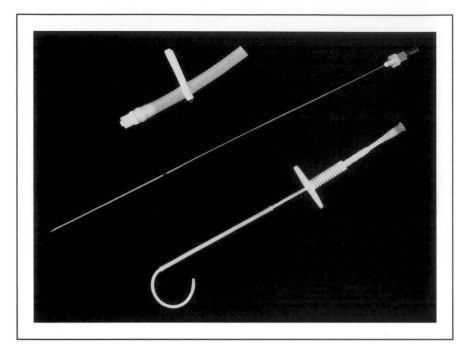

▲**Fig. 75** Paracentesis catheter. Normally used for suprapubic catheterisation, the catheter is easily introduced and when inserted its end curls up in the abdominal cavity. Fluid drains through side holes in the distal catheter.

Complications

Major

Peritoneal varices are rare but can be ruptured by the insertion of an ascitic drain. Severe haemorrhage after abdominal paracentesis occurs in 0.2% of patients with liver disease. This is more likely in those with severe liver failure or with significant renal dysfunction, but bleeding is not related to operator experience, elevated INR or low platelets.

Minor

- Failure to drain ascites: if the patient has had previous paracenteses the abdominal fluid often becomes loculated and the drain may need to be inserted under ultrasound guidance.

- Infection at exit site.

3.7 Liver biopsy

The aim is to obtain a core of liver tissue of sufficient length (about 2 cm, with six to eight portal tracts) to allow the histopathologist to establish a diagnosis. The procedure can be performed 'blind' without imaging at the bedside, ultrasound guided or via the transjugular route. There is a move away from 'blind' biopsies to all biopsies being ultrasound guided, which is probably associated with a higher success rate and less pain, although there is no evidence that significant life-threatening complications are reduced.

> Liver biopsy can be performed as a day case in patients without cirrhosis who have normal coagulation.

Indications

Indications for liver biopsy include acute hepatitis, drug-related hepatitis, chronic liver disease, cirrhosis, post liver transplantation, space-occupying lesions, unexplained hepatomegaly or liver enzyme elevations. Ultrasound-guided biopsy is specifically indicated in focal liver lesion, small liver or emphysema. Transjugular liver biopsy (Fig. 76) is specifically indicated in ascites, prolonged prothrombin time (PT) >4 seconds or a platelet count <60 × 10⁹/L.

Contraindications

A percutaneous liver biopsy is usually contraindicated where there is ascites, coagulopathy or an uncooperative patient.

Practical details

Details are for percutaneous non-radiologically guided liver biopsies. Note that an assistant is needed.

Before the procedure

Platelet count should be $>60 \times 10^9$/L and PT <3 seconds prolonged: if 3–4 seconds prolonged, give fresh frozen plasma just prior to procedure. Sedation is usually avoided as the patient has to cooperate with breathing, but if sedation is required then use midazolam with monitoring of oxygen saturations. If the patient has renal failure, then desmopressin acetate (DDAVP) should be given.

Equipment comprises the following:

- Menghini needle 1.9 mm diameter × 80–100 mm long (Fig. 77), or a Tru-cut needle;

- saline 10 mL;

- blade;

- lidocaine 1 or 2% (10 mL);

- needles for instillation of local anaesthetic;

- formalin in a sterile container.

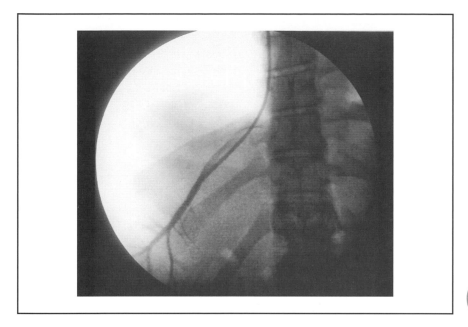

Fig. 76 Transjugular biopsy. Contrast is seen in a hepatic vein with the biopsy needle in the vein.

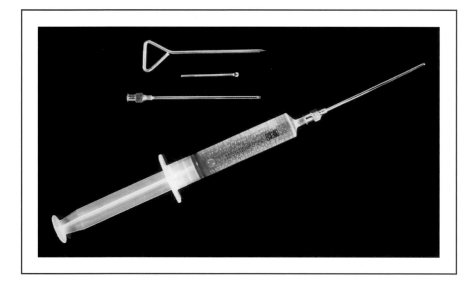

Fig. 77 Menghini biopsy needle.

If using the Menghini needle a cut is made in the skin. A track is then made down to the liver capsule using the metal needle in the Menghini pack. The biopsy is now performed by inserting the Menghini needle (attached to a syringe of saline) down the preformed track as far as the liver capsule. Then, while the patient is holding his or her breath in expiration, the needle is advanced quickly 2–3 cm in and out of the liver while continuously aspirating back on the syringe.

 No more than two passes into the liver should be made.

After the procedure

Ensure analgesia with paracetamol or codeine; narcotics are occasionally needed. The patient lies flat for 2 hours, with 6 hours bed-rest. BP and pulse recorded every 15 minutes for the first 2 hours and then half-hourly for 2 hours and then hourly.

Handling of specimens The tissue should go into formaldehyde for routine histology. If Wilson's disease is suspected, part of the biopsy is sent fresh for biochemical analysis. If tuberculosis is suspected, part of the biopsy should be placed in a sterile vial for microbiology.

Complications

Mortality rate is 0.01%.

Major

Haemorrhage occurs in 0.5%, usually in the first 3–4 hours post biopsy. There is a higher rate in malignancy and it is rare in the non-jaundiced patient. If there is major bleeding, angiography followed by transcatheter hepatic embolisation may be needed. Intrahepatic haematomas are rare, but may be

The procedure

Lie the patient flat on the back. Mark the first dull intercostal space on expiration in the mid-axillary line: the needle should be inserted over the top of a rib, avoiding the intercostal vessels below the rib. Clean the skin with antiseptic. Anaesthetise down to the liver capsule with lidocaine: do this by advancing the needle slowly perpendicular to the skin with the patient holding their breath in expiration. You will feel the needle pass through skin and muscle and over the rib, and you will hear it moving against the liver capsule when the patient breathes. It is important that you fully anaesthetise the liver capsule.

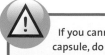 If you cannot identify the capsule, do not continue.

seen up to 24 hours after biopsy and should be considered if there is severe pain, fever or right upper quadrant tenderness. Pneumothorax/haemothorax are uncommon. Cholangitis can occur after a biopsy, particularly if there is underlying biliary disease, but it usually settles well with antibiotics.

Minor

A small amount of bleeding is universal and minor discomfort is common. Pain is more likely during and after the procedure if the capsule is inadequately anaesthetised.

FURTHER READING

Grant A, Neuberger J, Day C and Saxseena S (on behalf the British Society of Gastroenterology and the British Association for the Study of the Liver). *Guidelines on the Use of Liver Biopsy in Clinical Practice*. London: British Society for Gastroenterology, 2004. Full text available at http://www.bsg.org.uk/

4.1 Self-assessment questions

Question 1

Clinical scenario

A 24-year-old student with well-controlled ulcerative colitis treated with sulfasalazine and azathioprine develops acute diarrhoea during a brief visit to Thailand.

Question

Which is the most seriously *incorrect* response from the list below?

Answers

A The most likely diagnosis is an acute exacerbation of ulcerative colitis, which could be treated with a higher dose of sulfasalazine, or with oral or parenteral corticosteroids

B The most likely diagnosis is infectious diarrhoea, which could be treated with a course of antibiotics such as ciprofloxacin or metronidazole

C Long-term treatment with azathioprine might predispose the patient to opportunistic infection and broad-spectrum antimicrobial, antiviral, antiprotozoal and antifungal therapy might be indicated

D The likely diagnosis is acute exacerbation of ulcerative colitis or infectious diarrhoea, which could be treated with antidiarrhoeals such as codeine or loperamide, used judiciously for a short time to provide symptomatic relief

E The likely diagnosis is acute exacerbation of ulcerative colitis or infectious diarrhoea, which could be treated with a combination of antibiotics and oral corticosteroids, until a definitive diagnosis can be established

Question 2

Clinical scenario

A 50-year-old woman who is generally well apart from having troublesome osteoarthritis of the knees complains of profuse watery diarrhoea that has steadily worsened over the last 3 months.

Question

Select the most appropriate response from the list below:

Answers

A A full clinical evaluation, followed by blood tests and colonoscopy are probably required

B It is likely that this is an adverse event related to medications she might be taking, such as NSAIDs

C Watery diarrhoea with hypokalaemia, caused by a vasoactive intestinal peptide (VIP)-secreting tumour, is the likely diagnosis

D The progressive nature of the symptoms suggests a malignant process

E Microscopic colitis is the most likely diagnosis

Question 3

Clinical scenario

A 40-year-old man presents to your clinic with a history of alternating bouts of diarrhoea and constipation. He has no other significant symptoms, but his father was found to have colon cancer at the age of 70 years and he is anxious about the possibility that he may have early bowel cancer.

Question

Which two of the following statements are correct?

Answers

A The risk of colon cancer increases markedly after the age of 50 years

B Alternating constipation and diarrhoea are highly suspicious of neoplastic obstruction

C Screening for mutations in the *APC* and *HNPCC* genes has significantly altered the routine management of familial colon cancer

D A screening colonoscopy is a reasonable first step in the diagnostic algorithm, and should be arranged as soon as possible

E If the FBC and tumour markers are normal, there is little chance that he has colon cancer

F Faecal occult blood testing should be performed to exclude colon cancer

G It is likely that the patient's father has a sporadic form of colon cancer, and the patient is at no increased risk

H Annual colonoscopy is likely to be necessary if the patient is found to have adenomatous polyps

I Regular use of aspirin could halve the patient's risk of developing adenomatous polyps of the colon

J Regular use of folic acid supplements could halve the

patient's risk of developing adenomatous polyps of the colon

Question 4

Clinical scenario

A young white woman is referred for investigation of low BMI. She denies any gastrointestinal symptoms and seems generally quite healthy, although thin and with a BMI of 17.

Question

Which of the following statements is probably *not* correct?

Answers

A Coeliac disease is a cause of low body weight and may be asymptomatic

B Anorexia nervosa should be considered in the differential diagnosis

C Thyroid disease is unlikely and isolated biochemical abnormalities in the absence of symptoms should be interpreted with caution, as they can lead to over-diagnosis and treatment

D Crohn's disease is unlikely to cause low body weight unless it is very severe, when it is likely to be symptomatic

E Occult colorectal cancer is highly unlikely in this scenario

Question 5

Clinical scenario

You are devising a management algorithm to be used in a rapid-access, nurse-led clinic for patients complaining of dysphagia.

Question

Which of the following recommendations would you support?

Answers

A Patients with a history of weight loss and progressive dysphagia should be assessed urgently with a water-soluble contrast swallow

test, followed by upper endoscopy if indicated

B Empiric treatment with a proton pump inhibitor may be offered for up to 4 weeks

C Urgent upper endoscopy, biopsy and brushings should be arranged

D Achalasia is the most likely diagnosis in younger patients and the first test to be performed should be oesophageal manometry

E Peptic stricture secondary to acid reflux is the most likely diagnosis in middle-aged patients, and the first test to be performed should be 24-hour oesophageal pH monitoring

Question 6

Clinical scenario

A 70-year-old woman with pneumonia who has been treated with a third-generation cephalosporin develops profuse diarrhoea.

Question

Which of the following statements about her situation is correct?

Answers

A The patient is likely to have developed pseudomembranous colitis due to infection with *Clostridium difficile*

B Significant infection with *C. difficile* is associated with enterotoxin A, which can be rapidly detected by a sensitive ELISA test

C Rectal bleeding associated with diarrhoea makes it unlikely that it is related to the use of antibiotics

D Her antibiotic treatment should be broadened to include a fluoroquinolone such as ciprofloxacin to cover infection with dysentery-causing organisms

E The concurrent use of antibiotics means that it will be impossible to determine if her diarrhoea is

caused by infection with *C. difficile*

Question 7

Clinical scenario

A 20-year-old man with HIV infection develops profuse watery diarrhoea.

Question

Which of the following statements regarding HIV infection and the gastrointestinal tract is correct?

Answers

A HIV infects CD4-positive lymphocytes and is therefore minimally present in the gastrointestinal tract, which is predominantly populated with CD8-positive lymphocytes

B HIV infection reduces adaptive immunity by reducing the number of CD4-positive cells and therefore has minimal effects on intestinal immunity because it is mainly mediated by innate defence mechanisms

C Opportunistic infections such cryptosporidiosis are unlikely if the patient has a CD4-positive lymphocyte count >200 cells/mL

D The most likely cause of diarrhoea is an opportunistic infection, even if the patient's CD4-positive lymphocyte count is normal

E If the diarrhoea is profuse, there is a small risk of fecal–oral transmission of HIV infection to carers

Question 8

Clinical scenario

An obese patient reports to you that he has recently been following the Atkins diet, in which all forms of carbohydrate are avoided and subjects eat high-protein, high-fat meals.

Question

Which of the following statements is correct?

Answers

A It is unlikely that the subject will lose weight because of the high energy density of the foods consumed

B The long-term consequences of following this diet might include vitamin and micronutrient deficiency, dyslipidaemia, accelerated atherosclerosis and neoplasia

C The absence of carbohydrate in the diet results in significant hypoglycaemia

D The absence of carbohydrate in the diet inhibits the absorption of other nutrients, such as amino acids and triglycerides

E The diet has not been tested in clinical trials

Question 9

Clinical scenario

A 56-year-old woman presents to her GP with lethargy and tiredness. Her routine blood tests are normal apart from an alkaline phosphatase twice the upper limit of normal. Subsequent testing of liver antibodies show her to be positive for anti-mitochondrial antibody (M2 subtype).

Question

What should the patient be told?

Answers

A That she has primary biliary cirrhosis and will urgently need referral to a liver transplant unit

B That she has symptomatic primary biliary cirrhosis and will need a liver biopsy to stage her disease

C That she has primary biliary cirrhosis and will need follow-up in a liver clinic

D That no treatment is available for primary biliary cirrhosis

E That no further investigation or treatment will be needed

Question 10

Clinical scenario

A 25-year-old heavily pregnant woman returns to the UK from a holiday in Bangladesh where she visited family. Two weeks later she presents jaundiced and confused to casualty with an INR of 2, alanine transaminase (ALT) of 2,000 U/L and bilirubin of 200 µmol/L.

Question

Which viral infection is most likely to have caused this illness?

Answers

A Hepatitis A

B Hepatitis B

C Hepatitis C

D Hepatitis D

E Hepatitis E

Question 11

Clinical scenario

Prior to starting medical school, a prospective student is tested for hepatitis B. Her liver tests show alanine transaminase (ALT) 120 U/L and serology shows her to be positive for HBsAg, HBcAb and HBeAg, with a viral load of 10^5 genome equivalents/mL. A liver biopsy is reported as showing early fibrosis with evidence of moderate inflammation.

Question

Treatment should be offered to this patient in the form of:

Answers

A Interferon beta

B Interferon alfa 2b

C Pegylated interferon alfa 2a and ribavirin

D Basiliximab

E Entecavir

Question 12

Clinical scenario

An 18-year-old man admits to having taken 12 g of paracetamol 1 day prior to presentation in the Emergency Department with abdominal pain.

Question

Which of the following factors is most important in determining treatment?

Answers

A His paracetamol level

B His serum bilirubin

C His serum alanine transaminase

D His history

E His serum creatinine

Question 13

Clinical scenario

You are looking after a 35-year-old woman with a 10-year history of alcohol abuse (>50 units/week). She has been given a diagnosis of alcoholic hepatitis based on her history, and investigations show a bilirubin of 250 µmol/L, alanine transaminase (ALT) of 120 U/L and INR of 2. Her creatinine has increased over the last 2 days from 90 to 250 µmol/L.

Question

In managing her further which single investigation would be most helpful?

Answers

A Urine osmolality

B Urine microscopy

C Serum antineutrophil cytoplasmic antibody

D Creatinine clearance

E Spot urine sodium

Question 14

Clinical scenario

You are reviewing an 80-year-old man who presents to clinic with a 2-week history of jaundice, not associated with any pain. He feels lethargic but is otherwise well. Initial hepatitis serology is negative, ultrasound shows no duct dilatation, and liver function tests are cholestatic in nature. His medications have not changed over the last 2 years, apart from a recent course of Augmentin (co-amoxiclav) for cellulitis.

Question

Which of his medications may explain his jaundice?

Answers

A Atorvastatin
B Aspirin
C Augmentin (co-amoxiclav)
D Amiodarone
E Diclofenac

Question 15

Clinical scenario

A 35-year-old woman has an ultrasound scan for investigation of epigastic pain. Her liver function tests are all normal, and by the time of her scan her symptoms have abated on ranitidine. The report reads as follows: 'There are multiple small hyperechoic lesions in both lobes of the liver. No other focal lesions. No features to suggest cirrhosis or portal hypertension. Intrahepatic and extrahepatic biliary tree normal. Pancreas, kidneys, spleen normal.'

Question

The most likely diagnosis is:

Answers

A Multiple metastasis
B Focal nodular hyperplasia
C Adenomas
D Haemangiomas
E Liver abscesses

Question 16

Clinical scenario

You admit a 45-year-old man who had a liver transplant just over 3 months ago for primary sclerosing cholangitis. He complains of fever, abdominal pain and diarrhoea, which has come on over the last week. He has a platelet count of 60×10^9/L and alanine transaminase (ALT) of 300 U/L with a normal bilirubin. He is taking tacrolimus and prednisolone for immunosuppression. He tells you that he recently stopped taking valganciclovir.

Question

What is the most likely diagnosis?

Answers

A Acute rejection
B Chronic rejection
C Donor-acquired toxoplasmosis
D Donor-acquired cytomegalovirus
E Recurrence of his primary sclerosing cholangitis

Question 17

Clinical scenario

A 35-year-old woman, diagnosed 18 months previously with coeliac disease (biopsy-proven), now presents to outpatients with unresolved diarrhoea. Her bowels are open up to six times per day. There is no blood in the stools and she does not have abdominal pain.

Question

What are the two most useful tests to perform to investigate her diarrhoea?

Answers

A Lactose hydrogen breath test
B Repeat coeliac antibodies
C Repeat duodenal biopsy
D Colonoscopy
E Dietitian review
F Ultrasound of the abdomen
G Glucose hydrogen breath test

H Faecal elastase-1 level
I Thyroid function tests
J Small bowel meal

Question 18

Clinical scenario

A 45-year-old man presents with chronic epigastric pain radiating through to the back and steatorrhoea. He consumes 4–5 units of alcohol per week and has no family history of pancreatic disease. He has no other significant past medical history. CT scanning of the abdomen reveals a dilated pancreatic duct with associated calcification of the gland. Subsequent endoscopic retrograde cholangiopancreatography (ERCP) shows similar findings with no dominant structure. He is started on Creon (pancreatin) 3 tablets tds and there is improvement in his steatorrhoea.

Question

Which test might be helpful in determining the cause of his pancreatic disease?

Answers

A Magnetic resonance cholangiopancreatography (MRCP)
B Serum lipid profile
C Endoscopic ultrasound
D Serum amylase
E Pancreatic biopsy

Question 19

Clinical scenario

A 66-year-old woman is referred urgently with painless jaundice and weight loss. Bilirubin is 212 µmol/L, alanine transaminase (ALT) 60 U/L, alkaline phosphatase (ALP) 605 U/L, albumin 34 g/L and prothrombin time 17 seconds. Ultrasound scanning of the abdomen shows a grossly dilated biliary tree and a dilated pancreatic duct, but no mass is seen.

Question

What is the next most appropriate step in her management?

Answers

A Endoscopic retrograde cholangiopancreatography (ERCP)

B Abdominal CT scan

C Pancreatic endoscopic ultrasound

D Check CA19-9

E Laparoscopy

Question 20

Clinical scenario

A 30-year-old man is admitted with haemoglobin 5.2 g/dL, mean corpuscular volume 55.4 fL and ferritin 3 µg/L (normal range 14–200). B_{12} and folate levels are normal. He has had no haematemesis or malaena and no abdominal symptoms. An upper gastrointestinal endoscopy is performed. Figure 78 shows the appearance in the second part of the duodenum.

Question

What should be the next step in management?

Answers

A Sclerotherapy with alcohol and adrenaline

B Angiography and embolisation

C Thermal ablation with argon plasma coagulation

D Application of endoscopic bands

E Biopsy

Question 21

Clinical scenario

A 40-year-old woman presents to the outpatient clinic with intermittent epigastric discomfort. FBC, urea and electrolytes are normal. Liver function tests reveal alkaline phosphatase (ALP) 600 U/L, γ-glutamyltransferase (GGT) 768 U/L, bilirubin 13 µmol/L,

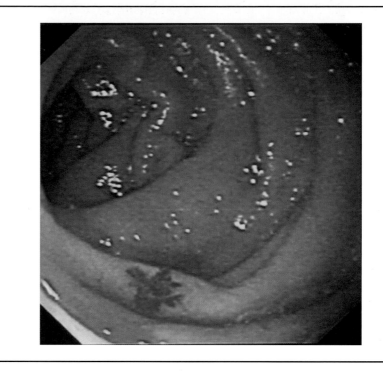

▲ **Fig. 78** Question 20.

alanine transaminase (ALT) 26 U/L and albumin 39 g/L. Transabdominal ultrasound shows normal liver architecture, but there are several small stones in the gallbladder and the common bile duct measures 10 mm in diameter. The pancreas and the main pancreatic duct are normal.

Question

What would be the most appropriate next step?

Answers

A Endoscopic retrograde cholangiopancreatography and bile duct trawl

B CT scan

C CA19-9

D Magnetic resonance cholangiopancreatography (MRCP)

E Refer for laparoscopic cholecystectomy and bile duct exploration

Question 22

Clinical scenario

A 79-year-old man presents with obstructive jaundice and is found to have a non-resectable adenocarcinoma of the pancreatic head. The decision at the multidisciplinary team meeting is that he should receive palliative care and that his jaundice should be relieved by inserting a biliary stent.

Question

Which of the following factors would favour stent insertion via percutaneous transhepatic cholangiography (PTC) rather than endoscopic retrograde cholangiopancreatography (ERCP)?

Answers

A Prothrombin time of 17 seconds

B Presence of ascites

C Underlying chronic liver disease

D Platelet count of 70×10^9/L

E Previous Polya gastrectomy

Question 23

Clinical scenario

A 48-year-old man with type 1 diabetes mellitus of 8 years' duration attends outpatients with a history of opening his bowels five to six times per day over the last 6 months. There is no blood or mucus in the stool and he has not had any abdominal pain. His HbA_{1c} is 7.0%. FBC, urea and electrolytes, liver function tests, thyroid function tests, abdominal ultrasound and colonoscopy with random biopsies are all normal.

Question

Which two of the following tests are most likely to lead to a diagnosis?

Answers

A Autonomic function tests
B *Helicobacter* serology
C Stool for microscopy, culture and sensitivity
D Abdominal CT scan
E Small bowel enema
F Stool for faecal elastase
G Lactose hydrogen breath test
H Small bowel manometry
I Glycocholate hydrogen breath test
J Rigid sigmoidoscopy and rectal deep rectal biopsy

Question 24

Clinical scenario

A 40-year-old man is referred with a 12-month history of diarrhoea.

Question

Which one of the following features would be *against* a diagnosis of irritable bowel syndrome?

Answers

A Passage of mucus with the motions.
B Nocturnal diarrhoea

C Abdominal discomfort relieved by defecation
D Abdominal bloating
E Onset of symptoms following an episode of *Campylobacter* diarrhoea

Question 25

Clinical scenario

A 66-year-old man is referred to the gastroenterology outpatient clinic for investigation of a 6-month history of diarrhoea.

Question

Which two of the following statements are true?

Answers

A Colonoscopic investigation should only be offered if alert symptoms such as weight loss or rectal bleeding are present
B Rigid sigmoidoscopy and rectal biopsy will exclude microscopic colitis
C Normal inflammatory markers (ESR/CRP) do not exclude inflammatory bowel disease as a cause of his symptoms
D Coeliac antibodies should only be performed if the patient gives a history of symptoms worsening on exposure to wheat
E Crohn's disease is an unlikely diagnosis in a man of his age
F A history of cholecystectomy preceding the onset of his symptoms may suggest a diagnosis of microscopic colitis
G The presence of abdominal pain is highly suggestive of ulcerative colitis
H Colorectal cancer is a possible diagnosis
I Nocturnal diarrhoea is common in the elderly
J Peptic ulceration is a likely cause

4.2 Self-assessment answers

Answer to Question 1

D

Acute diarrhoea is usually infectious in aetiology, although other causes such as medications, food intolerance and inflammatory bowel disease (IBD) need to be considered. In patients with a known history of IBD it is often difficult to distinguish an exacerbation of disease activity from an infectious gastroenteritis, and it is pragmatic to treat for both until the diagnosis can be established, which often cannot be achieved with any certainty. Symptomatic treatment with antidiarrhoeals can be highly dangerous because it can both mask the severity of the illness and potentially aggravate it by inhibiting the excretion of pathogens. Azathioprine is used at a relatively low dose in IBD and is unlikely to cause life-threatening immunosuppression unless there is severe myelosuppression, which may develop after months and/or years of uneventful treatment; hence patients on thiopurine treatment should have regular FBC.

Answer to Question 2

A

Chronic diarrhoea may be due to a large number of different causes, hence a full evaluation of patients presenting in this way is mandatory. This patient may well have used NSAIDs that are associated with the development of microscopic or lymphocytic colitis, which is a typical cause of watery diarrhoea in middle-aged and elderly women.

However, without a full history, examination and supportive investigations, this possibility is not necessarily highly or most likely. VIPoma is exceedingly rare, and there is no evidence in favour of a malignant process in this patient.

Answer to Question 3

A, F

Colorectal cancer is the third commonest cause of cancer-related death, and the lifetime risk of developing the condition is about 1 in 50. However, this risk is very low in early life and rises steeply after the age of 50 years. Typically, colorectal cancer may be asymptomatic or it may present with constipation, diarrhoea, rectal bleeding, abdominal pain, unexplained iron deficiency or anaemia. Alternating constipation and diarrhoea, especially if long-standing, is more indicative of irritable bowel syndrome.

Germline mutations in the *APC* gene are exceedingly rare, although when they occur, they cause an autosomally dominant form of hereditary colorectal cancer. Hereditary non-polyposis colon cancer (HNPCC) is a clinical syndrome describing an inherited tendency to develop cancer without a preceding history of adenomatous polyps. It is associated with mutations in a number of different genes, particularly those associated with correcting defects in DNA replication at the cellular level (mismatch-repair genes). Genetic testing for HNPCC is complex and not easily applied in clinical practice.

Even in cases of apparently sporadic colorectal cancer there is probably an increased risk in first-degree relatives, probably as a consequence of genetic and environmental factors such as diet. Strategies for screening the population at risk for colorectal cancer are evolving and are currently focused on those older than 50 years, or in cases of familial cancer at an age 10 years younger than the youngest affected family member. In these cases, faecal occult blood testing followed by sigmoidoscopy or colonoscopy, or colonoscopy on its own, at 5-yearly intervals are favoured options.

Use of NSAIDs and aspirin significantly slows the development of adenomatous polyps, which are the precursors of colorectal cancer, although the relative benefit may be offset by an increased risk of intestinal bleeding due to peptic ulceration. Folic acid has no proven effect.

Answer to Question 4

C

Low body weight or weight loss may be caused by many processes, including dietary habits, exercise, smoking and undiagnosed medical illnesses such as coeliac disease, Crohn's disease and thyrotoxicosis. The symptoms and signs of these conditions may be very mild, and with an insidious onset the patient may complain of few or no symptoms at all. This is most true for coeliac disease and hyperthyroidism, which might only be detected by special tests (coeliac serology and thyroid function tests). Crohn's disease is unlikely to cause significant weight loss without also causing abdominal pain and diarrhoea, which might be mistaken for symptoms of irritable bowel syndrome. At this age, occult colorectal cancer is highly unlikely.

Answer to Question 5

A

A barium swallow should be obtained before endoscopy in patients presenting with symptoms of oesophageal obstruction to provide guidance to the endoscopist and to avoid inadvertent perforation of a malignant lesion. Patients with oesophageal obstruction are at risk of aspiration pneumonia, which might be reduced by using a water-soluble contrast medium rather than barium. Empiric acid suppression may be appropriate for simple reflux symptoms but is inappropriate when patients complain of difficulty swallowing, which may be due to malignant or benign stricturing, or dysmotility of the oesophagus. Physiological tests such as manometry and pH monitoring can help to refine the diagnosis, but they are best used after more common or serious conditions have been excluded.

Answer to Question 6

B

Antibiotic-associated diarrhoea frequently develops after use of broad-spectrum antibiotics. In many cases it is not associated with toxigenic *C. difficile* infection and may clear simply on withdrawal of the antibiotics. Significant *C. difficile* infection is associated with production by the bacteria of enterotoxins, which can be rapidly detected in the stool using tests such as ELISA. Detection of *C. difficile* infection is not compromised by concurrent use of antibiotics. In severe cases, toxigenic *C. difficile* infection can cause pseudomembranous colitis, which is associated with the passage of blood and mucus per rectum. In these cases the appropriate first line of treatment is withdrawal of broad-spectrum antibiotics if possible, and administration of metronidazole or oral vancomycin.

Answer to Question 7

C

There is increasing evidence that HIV infection has profound effects on the gastrointestinal immune system, despite the relative predominance of CD8-positive T lymphocytes in this compartment. Patients on long-term antiretroviral treatment may harbour a reservoir of infection in the intestine that allows reactivation when medications are withdrawn. Defence mechanisms in the intestine are critically dependent on the function of T lymphocytes, including a specialised group of intraepithelial lymphocytes confined to the intestine. Opportunistic intestinal infections are rare when the CD count is satisfactory and more frequent when the count is low. Despite the high levels of virus in gastrointestinal secretions, including saliva, HIV does not seem to infect via the oral route, although infection by rectal, vaginal and parenteral routes occurs readily.

Answer to Question 8

B

Anecdotal reports and clinical studies demonstrate that ketogenic diets such as the Atkins diet can lead to substantial loss of weight. This probably occurs through ketogenic metabolism of fat and suppression of appetite by the high intake of protein. The relative paucity of carbohydrate in the diet is unlikely to affect the absorption of other nutrients, although the lack of fruit, vegetables and starchy foods may lead to deficiencies of calcium, iron, folate and other vitamins. With the paucity of glucose in the diet, blood levels can be maintained by gluconeogenesis. The relatively high intake of fats and red meat and low intake of vitamins and fibre may predispose to atherogenesis and colorectal cancer.

Answer to Question 9

C

Primary biliary cirrhosis (PBC) is a disease characterised by inflammatory destruction of the small bile ducts within the liver, eventually leading to cirrhosis of the liver. The cause of PBC is unknown, but because of the presence of autoantibodies it is generally thought to be an autoimmune disease. In the presence of typical symptoms, liver enzyme abnormalities and positive M2 anti-mitochondrial antibodies, the diagnosis can confidently be made without a liver biopsy. Most patients with PBC do not come to liver transplantation, which is reserved for those with documented decompensated liver disease or (very occasionally) uncontrollable symptoms (usually pruritus). In symptomatic patients ursodeoxycholic acid prolongs survival, and because of this – along with the need for surveillance for progressive liver disease – patients should have ongoing follow-up, usually performed by their local gastroenterologist/hepatologist.

Answer to Question 10

E

Infective hepatitis can be caused by a variety of different viruses such as hepatitis A, B, C, D and E. The incubation period following exposure to hepatitis E ranges from 3 to 8 weeks, with a mean of 40 days. Hepatitis E is usually a self-limiting infection followed by complete recovery; prolonged viraemia or faecal shedding is unusual and there is no chronic infection. A fulminant form of hepatitis E can develop, most frequently in pregnancy and with a mortality rate of 20% in the third trimester. The condition should therefore be suspected in outbreaks of water-borne hepatitis occurring in developing countries, especially if the disease is more severe in pregnant women, or if hepatitis A has been excluded. A correct diagnosis can only be made by testing for the presence of specific viral antigens and/or antiviral antibodies (with or without polymerase chain reaction for active viral replication).

Answer to Question 11

B

Government estimates are that about 180,000 people in the UK have chronic hepatitis B and the prevalence of hepatitis B surface antigen (HBsAg) among blood donors is around 1 in 1,500. Around one-fifth of HBsAg-positive individuals are HBeAg positive, with 7–20% spontaneously losing HBeAg positivity per year.

There are five therapies for chronic hepatitis B that are currently approved: interferon alfa-2b, lamivudine, adefovir, entecavir and pegylated interferon (peginterferon) alfa-2a. Given the need for long-term treatment, current guidelines recommend treatment only for patients with elevated aminotransferase levels or histological evidence of moderate or severe inflammation or advanced fibrosis. For patients with HBeAg-positive chronic hepatitis B who do not yet have cirrhosis, the goal is to achieve HBeAg seroconversion, and interferon alfa alone has the best chance of achieving this. Viral suppression without HBeAg clearance is invariably associated with relapse, whereas viral suppression with HBeAg clearance is associated with sustained responses in 50–90% of patients.

Students found to be infected with a blood-borne virus such as hepatitis B are allowed to continue their medical course leading to full medical registration provided they accept the requirement that they will not be allowed to perform exposure-prone procedures while infectious (HBeAg positive or HBeAg negative with >10^3 genome equivalents/mL HBV DNA), and that careers in some specialties may not be open to them. Registered medical students who are HBeAg negative and who have virus loads that do not exceed 10^3 genome equivalents/mL will be tested annually in order to confirm that their virus load has not exceeded the threshold at which they would be prohibited from conducting exposure-prone procedures. Those who have undergone a course of treatment need to show that they have a viral load that does not exceed 10^3 genome equivalents/mL 1 year after cessation of treatment before a return to unrestricted working practices can be considered.

Answer to Question 12

D

The history is most important in determining the risk of hepatotoxicity: a dose of paracetamol of as little as 75 mg/kg in someone at risk can be fatal. Risk factors include:

- regular ethanol consumption in excess of 21 units/week in males and 14 units/week in females;

- regular use of enzyme-inducing drugs (carbamazepine, phenytoin, phenobarbital, rifampacin);

- conditions causing glutathione depletion (malnutrition, HIV, eating disorders, cystic fibrosis).

In all scenarios you are strongly advised to treat with *N*-acetylcysteine if in doubt.

Answer to Question 13

E

Although not diagnostic, a low spot urinary sodium (<5 mmol/L) is in keeping with a diagnosis of hepatorenal syndrome (HRS), assuming that the patient does not have intravascular volume depletion. HRS is defined as an acute, functional and progressive reduction in renal blood flow and glomerular filtration rate (GFR) secondary to intense renal cortical vasoconstriction in the setting of decompensated liver disease. Other aetiologies for renal failure in liver disease must be excluded. HRS can be classified as type 1, with a rapidly progressive decline in GFR (<2 weeks), or type 2, which is not as rapidly progressive (>2 weeks).

Answer to Question 14

C

Virtually all drugs can cause liver injury. In this case the most recently introduced medication is most likely to be the cause of liver injury, assuming other investigations for chronic liver disease are negative. The prescription drugs to be particularly aware of when assessing a patient with an undiagnosed liver disorder include Augmentin (co-amoxiclav), diclofenac, isoniazid, erythromycin, sodium valproate, amiodarone and phenytoin.

Answer to Question 15

D

Liver imaging must always be interpreted in the context of the clinical information, particularly the presence or absence of relevant symptoms, the presence or absence

of liver function test abnormalities, and the presence or absence of cirrhosis. Liver masses with typical imaging features of simple cyst or haemangioma in patients not known to have, or not suspected of having, a malignancy may be classified as benign.

Haemangiomas, the commonest of the focal benign liver lesions, arise from the endothelial cells that line the blood vessels and consist of multiple large vascular channels lined by a single layer of endothelial cells and supported by collagenous walls. They are more common in women and occur at all ages, but most frequently in the third, fourth and fifth decades of life. Most are seen incidentally and are usually less than 1 cm in diameter. They are generally asymptomatic, although if large (>5 cm) may cause symptoms/signs such as pain, nausea or enlargement of the liver; very rarely they can rupture, causing severe pain and bleeding into the abdomen, or become infected. On ultrasound imaging hepatic haemangiomas are hyperechoic in 60–70% of cases, hypoechoic in 20% of cases, and have a mixed pattern with discrete margins in 20%; they are multiple in 10% of cases.

Answer to Question 16

D

Cytomegalovirus (CMV) infection is an important consideration in any organ transplant recipient, particularly where the recipient has never had infection but the donor is a carrier, since the recipient is then at risk of primary infection. For this reason close attention is given to prophylaxis, particularly in the first 3 months after transplantation. When prophylaxis is stopped there is still a chance of infection, which in the case of liver transplant recipients will often present as fever, abdominal pain, diarrhoea (colitis), breathlessness (pneumonitis) and hepatitis. Other features of the illness can include haematological abnormalities, retinitis and oesophagitis. Diagnosis is by quantifying CMV viraemia in the blood. Treatment is with intravenous ganciclovir and reduction of immunosuppression if possible.

Answer to Question 17

E, H

The most common cause of ongoing gastrointestinal symptoms in patients with coeliac disease is continued gluten exposure. Dietitians are best equipped to assess this and therefore should be involved in assessment. Up to 30% of patients with coeliac disease and unresolved diarrhoea have associated exocrine pancreatic insufficiency. The faecal elastase-1 test is cheap, non-invasive and simple to use in an outpatient setting. Positive coeliac antibodies may suggest continued gluten exposure but are not diagnostic. Repeat duodenal biopsy may still show villous atrophy even in compliant patients. Colonoscopy in a patient under 45 years is unlikely to demonstrate a significant cause for diarrhoea. Although thyroid disease is associated with coeliac disease and should be screened for, only 1–2% of patients develop new thyroid dysfunction over a 12-month period.

Answer to Question 18

B

Chronic pancreatitis is most commonly caused by alcohol but this man consumes only small quantities. MRCP may help to exclude obstructive causes or

congenital abnormalities, but ERCP and CT scan did not reveal either of these. Endoscopic ultrasound is unlikely to demonstrate the cause of pancreatitis at this stage. Pancreatic biopsy will show evidence of chronic pancreatitis but is unlikely to reveal the aetiology. It is possible that his pancreatitis may be caused by hyperlipidaemia.

Answer to Question 19

B

This scenario is highly suspicious of cancer in the pancreatic head as there is obstructive jaundice and ultrasound demonstrates the 'double duct' sign. The absence of a mass on ultrasound does not exclude this diagnosis and therefore a CT scan is required to further image the pancreatic head and simultaneously stage the disease. ERCP would demonstrate the stricture but gives no staging information, and endoscopic ultrasound may not pick up liver metastases. CA19-9 is not specific for pancreatic cancer and is often raised in obstructive jaundice of any aetiology. Laparoscopy is too invasive at this stage without further imaging.

Answer to Question 20

C

This is duodenal angiodysplasia and very likely to be the source of blood loss in this patient. It can be dealt with directly by applying argon electrocoagulation, with minimal time added to the procedure. Sclerotherapy and banding techniques are not appropriate for such a lesion. Angiography may not identify this lesion if it is not actively bleeding and embolisation may not be possible. Biopsy is hazardous as it may lead to torrential bleeding.

Answer to Question 21

D

As this woman is not acutely ill, there is time to perform further investigations of the biliary tree without moving directly to invasive procedures. MRCP has a higher sensitivity than CT for detecting distal bile duct stones, which are the most likely cause of this woman's presentation. CA19-9 is useless in this situation. If her MRCP is negative, then laparoscopic removal of the gallbladder would be appropriate.

Answer to Question 22

E

ERCP is usually preferable to PTC for insertion of biliary stents, unless ERCP has previously failed or there is altered anatomy. Patients who have had a Billroth II gastrectomy have grossly different anatomy and ERCP can be impossible to perform. Impaired clotting (raised prothrombin time, low platelets or liver disease) are contraindications to a percutaneous approach, as is the presence of ascites.

Answer to Question 23

F, I

The three most likely associations with type 1 diabetes mellitus that cause diarrhoea are coeliac disease (up to 5%, so check coeliac serology), exocrine pancreatic insufficiency (over 30% in some studies) and small bowel bacterial overgrowth (SBBO). SBBO commonly occurs when there is autonomic dysfunction, but tests of the autonomic nervous system may be normal, and SBBO may not be present in those with dysfunction. This patient also has good metabolic control of his diabetes as judged by HbA_{1c} of 7.0%. It will be appropriate to send stool for microscopy, culture and sensitivity, but after a history of 6 months this is likely to be normal. CT scanning or small bowel imaging will have a low yield. Lactose hydrogen breath testing may be falsely positive due to SBBO. Further colonic biopsies are unlikely to add anything.

Answer to Question 24

B

The Rome II diagnostic criteria for irritable bowel syndrome require the presence of abdominal pain for 12 weeks (not necessarily consecutive) with two of the following: relieved by defecation; onset associated with change in form of stool; onset associated with change in frequency of stool. Associated features may include the passage of mucus and the presence of abdominal bloating. Postinfectious irritable bowel syndrome is well recognised after an episode of culture-positive gastroenteritis. The presence of nocturnal diarrhoea or pain, weight loss, or abnormalities on blood tests should alert the physician to the possibility of inflammatory bowel disease or other organic disease.

Answer to Question 25

C, H

All patients over the age of 50 years with a persistent change in bowel habit should undergo colonoscopy (or double-contrast barium enema) to exclude colonic neoplasm. Rectal biopsies alone do not exclude microscopic colitis: it is recommended that biopsies are taken from the right and left colon. Mild or limited (eg proctitis) ulcerative colitis may present with normal inflammatory markers. Coeliac antibodies should be routinely performed in any patient with chronic diarrhoea. Many patients with irritable bowel syndrome exhibit intolerance to wheat. Crohn's disease has a bimodal distribution, with peaks between 15–40 years and 60–70 years. Cholecystectomy is associated with bile salt malabsorption. Abdominal pain is commonly seen in Crohn's disease but should alert the physician to complications in ulcerative colitis. Nocturnal diarrhoea should always be aggressively investigated as this is not a feature of functional disease.

THE MEDICAL MASTERCLASS SERIES

Clinical Skills

CLINICAL SKILLS FOR PACES

PAIN RELIEF AND PALLIATIVE CARE

MEDICINE FOR THE ELDERLY

Haematology and Oncology

HAEMATOLOGY

Cardiology and Respiratory Medicine

CARDIOLOGY

RESPIRATORY MEDICINE

Gastroenterology and Hepatology

GASTROENTEROLOGY AND HEPATOLOGY

Neurology, Ophthalmology and Psychiatry

NEUROLOGY

Endocrinology

ENDOCRINOLOGY

Nephrology

NEPHROLOGY

Rheumatology and Clinical Immunology

RHEUMATOLOGY AND CLINICAL IMMUNOLOGY

INDEX

Note: page numbers in *italics* refer to figures, those in **bold** refer to tables.